Redesigning the Process for Establishing the *Dietary Guidelines for Americans*

Committee to Review the Process to Update the
Dietary Guidelines for Americans

Food and Nutrition Board

Health and Medicine Division

A Consensus Study Report of

The National Academies of
SCIENCES · ENGINEERING · MEDICINE

THE NATIONAL ACADEMIES PRESS
Washington, DC
www.nap.edu

THE NATIONAL ACADEMIES PRESS 500 Fifth Street, NW Washington, DC 20001

This activity was supported by Contract No. AG-3198-C-16-0004 from the U.S. Department of Agriculture. Any opinions, findings, conclusions, or recommendations expressed in this publication do not necessarily reflect the views of any organization or agency that provided support for the project.

International Standard Book Number-13: 978-0-309-46482-6
International Standard Book Number-10: 0-309-46482-X
Digital Object Identifier: https://doi.org/10.17226/24883

Additional copies of this publication are available for sale from the National Academies Press, 500 Fifth Street, NW, Keck 360, Washington, DC 20001; (800) 624-6242 or (202) 334-3313; http://www.nap.edu.

Printed in the United States of America

Suggested citation: National Academies of Sciences, Engineering, and Medicine. 2017. *Redesigning the process for establishing the* Dietary Guidelines for Americans. Washington, DC: The National Academies Press. doi: https://doi.org/10.17226/24883.

The National Academies of

SCIENCES · ENGINEERING · MEDICINE

The **National Academy of Sciences** was established in 1863 by an Act of Congress, signed by President Lincoln, as a private, nongovernmental institution to advise the nation on issues related to science and technology. Members are elected by their peers for outstanding contributions to research. Dr. Marcia McNutt is president.

The **National Academy of Engineering** was established in 1964 under the charter of the National Academy of Sciences to bring the practices of engineering to advising the nation. Members are elected by their peers for extraordinary contributions to engineering. Dr. C. D. Mote, Jr., is president.

The **National Academy of Medicine** (formerly the Institute of Medicine) was established in 1970 under the charter of the National Academy of Sciences to advise the nation on medical and health issues. Members are elected by their peers for distinguished contributions to medicine and health. Dr. Victor J. Dzau is president.

The three Academies work together as the **National Academies of Sciences, Engineering, and Medicine** to provide independent, objective analysis and advice to the nation and conduct other activities to solve complex problems and inform public policy decisions. The National Academies also encourage education and research, recognize outstanding contributions to knowledge, and increase public understanding in matters of science, engineering, and medicine.

Learn more about the National Academies of Sciences, Engineering, and Medicine at **www.nationalacademies.org.**

The National Academies of
SCIENCES • ENGINEERING • MEDICINE

Consensus Study Reports published by the National Academies of Sciences, Engineering, and Medicine document the evidence-based consensus on the study's statement of task by an authoring committee of experts. Reports typically include findings, conclusions, and recommendations based on information gathered by the committee and the committee's deliberations. Each report has been subjected to a rigorous and independent peer-review process and it represents the position of the National Academies on the statement of task.

Proceedings published by the National Academies of Sciences, Engineering, and Medicine chronicle the presentations and discussions at a workshop, symposium, or other event convened by the National Academies. The statements and opinions contained in proceedings are those of the participants and are not endorsed by other participants, the planning committee, or the National Academies.

For information about other products and activities of the National Academies, please visit www.nationalacademies.org/about/whatwedo.

COMMITTEE TO REVIEW THE PROCESS TO UPDATE THE *DIETARY GUIDELINES FOR AMERICANS*

ROBERT M. RUSSELL (*Chair*), Professor Emeritus, Nutrition and Medicine, Tufts University School of Medicine, Boston, Massachusetts

JAMY ARD, Professor, Department of Epidemiology and Prevention; Co-Director, Wake Forest Baptist Health Weight Management Center, Wake Forest University Baptist Medical Center, Winston-Salem, North Carolina

STEPHANIE A. ATKINSON, Professor, Pediatrics, McMaster University, Hamilton, Ontario

CAROL J. BOUSHEY, Associate Researcher, Professor, Cancer Epidemiology Program; Director, Nutrition Support Shared Resource, University of Hawaii Cancer Center, Honolulu

SUSAN M. KREBS-SMITH, Chief, Risk Factor Assessment Branch, Epidemiology and Genomics Research Program, Division of Cancer Control and Population Sciences, National Cancer Institute, Bethesda, Maryland

JOSEPH LAU, Professor Emeritus, Center for Evidence Synthesis in Health, Department of Health Services, Policy & Practice, Brown University School of Public Health, Providence, Rhode Island

BRUCE Y. LEE, Director, Operations Research, International Vaccine Access Center; Executive Director, Global Obesity Prevention Center; Associate Professor, International Health, Johns Hopkins Bloomberg School of Public Health, Baltimore, Maryland

JOANNE R. LUPTON, Distinguished Professor Emerita, Texas A&M University, College Station

SALLY C. MORTON, Dean, College of Science, Virginia Tech, Blacksburg

NICOLAAS P. PRONK, President, HealthPartners Institute; Chief Science Officer, HealthPartners, Minneapolis, Minnesota

SUSAN B. ROBERTS, Director, Energy Metabolism Laboratory and Professor of Nutrition, U.S. Department of Agriculture Human Nutrition Research Center on Aging at Tufts University; Professor of Psychiatry and Staff Member in Pediatrics, Tufts Medical School, Boston, Massachusetts

A. CATHARINE ROSS, Professor, Nutrition and Physiology; Dorothy Foehr Chair and Professor, Department of Nutritional Sciences, The Pennsylvania State University, University Park

---

NOTE: See Appendix G, Disclosure of Conflicts of Interest.

BARBARA O. SCHNEEMAN, Emeritus Professor of Nutrition, Department of Nutrition and Department of Food Science and Technology, University of California, Davis
MARTÍN J. SEPÚLVEDA, IBM Fellow, Retired IBM Vice President of Health Systems and Policy Research, Watson Research Laboratory, IBM Corporation, St. Augustine, Florida

Health and Medicine Division Study Staff

SAMANTHA M. CHAO, Study Director
MEGHAN E. QUIRK, Senior Program Officer
MEREDITH J. YOUNG, Senior Program Assistant
ANNA BURY, Research Associate
ANN L. YAKTINE, Director, Food and Nutrition Board

Reviewers

This Consensus Study Report was reviewed in draft form by individuals chosen for their diverse perspectives and technical expertise. The purpose of this independent review is to provide candid and critical comments that will assist the National Academies of Sciences, Engineering, and Medicine in making each published report as sound as possible and to ensure that it meets the institutional standards for quality, objectivity, evidence, and responsiveness to the study charge. The review comments and draft manuscript remain confidential to protect the integrity of the deliberative process.

We thank the following individuals for their review of this report:

CHERYL ACHTERBERG, The Ohio State University
ALICIA CARRIQUIRY, Iowa State University
WILLIAM H. DIETZ, The George Washington University
CHRISTINA ECONOMOS, Tufts University
JOHN W. ERDMAN, JR., University of Illinois at Urbana-Champaign
PETER BARTON HUTT, Covington & Burling LLP
RONALD M. KRAUSS, Children's Hospital Oakland Research Institute and University of California, San Francisco
PENNY KRIS-ETHERTON, The Pennsylvania State University
SUZANNE P. MURPHY, Emeritus, University of Hawaii Cancer Center
ESTHER F. MYERS, EF Myers Consulting, Inc.
DEBORAH L. O'CONNOR, University of Toronto

ROBERT C. POST, Chobani Nutrition Center, Chobani, LLC, and formerly with the U.S. Department of Agriculture Center for Nutrition Policy and Promotion
HOLGER J. SCHÜNEMANN, McMaster University
PAUL SHEKELLE, RAND Corporation
PATRICK J. STOVER, Cornell University

Although the reviewers listed above provided many constructive comments and suggestions, they were not asked to endorse the conclusions or recommendations of this report nor did they see the final draft before its release. The review of this report was overseen by **SUE CURRY,** University of Iowa, and **JOHANNA T. DWYER,** Tufts Medical Center. They were responsible for making certain that an independent examination of this report was carried out in accordance with the standards of the National Academies and that all review comments were carefully considered. Responsibility for the final content rests entirely with the authoring committee and the National Academies.

Preface

This is the second and final installment of a report that examines and then suggests improvements for the entire process used for establishing the *Dietary Guidelines for Americans* (*DGA*). This report is a consensus product of a committee of the National Academies of Sciences, Engineering, and Medicine as mandated by Congress in the Consolidated Appropriations Act of 2016. The first report was released in February 2017 and suggested changes to be made in the selection process of members of the Dietary Guidelines Advisory Committee (DGAC). In this report, the DGAC is called the DGSAC to stand for the Dietary Guidelines Scientific Advisory Committee. This second report focuses on a process redesign in developing and updating the guidelines, beyond just the selection of members for the DGSAC. This National Academies committee was specifically asked to evaluate the process, but *not* to evaluate the content, recommendations, or scientific justifications used in the current or past editions of the *DGA*.

Over time, the role of the *DGA* has become two-fold: (1) they provide the public with science-based dietary advice on eating patterns that can help to reduce the risk of developing a chronic disease, and (2) they provide food-based guidance (types and composition of foods to be used) in federal nutrition programs, such as the National School Lunch Program, the Special Supplemental Nutrition Program for Women, Infants, and Children (WIC) program, and many others. Despite the huge amount of effort that goes into establishing the *DGA*, less than 10 percent of Americans actually follow the guidelines. Congress has suggested that the low level of adherence could be the result of a lack of confidence, in part because of how the *DGA* have been developed and hence a low level of trust in the ultimate recommendations. Congress thus directed the U.S. Department of Agriculture (USDA) to engage the National Academies to establish this ad hoc committee to conduct a comprehensive evaluation of the processes used to establish the *DGA*. (The Statement of Task can be found in the Introduction in Box 1-3.)

A principal finding of this National Academies committee is that an inefficiency of effort and a lack of continuity exists between successive 5-year *DGA* cycles. Within a 5-year cycle, the current process allots 2 years for evaluation of the science and for making conclusions by the DGAC, and 1 year for developing the *DGA Policy Report* by the government. The remaining 2 years of the 5-year cycle are a period of relative inactivity. This National Academies committee believes that using the entire 5 years for work on the *DGA* will not only provide the opportunity for a more thorough evaluation of the science, but also allow the *DGA* process to become more agile, flexible, and effective—and will address more topics of interest to the general public.

Currently, topic identification, gathering of scientific data, and the synthesis and interpretation of the science all fall on the shoulders of a single DGAC to be completed within a 2-year time frame. A central recommendation of this National Academies committee is to allow for more focused and tailored groups of experts to undertake each of the functions by dividing them among several groups during the 5-year cycle. The division of functions and the use of the entire 5-year time period for work on the *DGA* would provide many more opportunities for stakeholder and public participation, and thus serve to insert greater transparency into the process. If the *DGA* omits or only accepts parts of the conclusions in the DGSAC report, a clear explanation has to be given as to why. We believe these steps would all contribute to a higher degree of integrity and thus enhance the trustworthiness of the process to develop the *DGA* (see Recommendations 1 and 2).

Our National Academies committee also believes it is critical that the methods used to inform the *DGA* be validated and appropriate to the questions being asked. After extensive evaluation, we found that the current methods being used in the *DGA* process—original systematic reviews; existing systematic reviews, meta-analyses, and reports; food pattern modeling; and descriptive data analysis—are indeed appropriate. However, the vetting and updating of methods could be greatly strengthened by putting out the systematic reviews done at USDA's Nutritional Evidence Library (NEL) for external peer review before handing them over to the DGSAC (see Recommendation 3). Moreover, there should be ongoing evaluation of NEL methods and ongoing training of NEL staff by external expert groups with greater investment made in supportive, technological infrastructure (see Recommendation 4).

The final three recommendations made by this National Academies committee (see Recommendations 5, 6, and 7) are for strengthening and adopting appropriate and strategic methodologies so as always to align with current best practices. Scientific methods are continually evolving as new ones are emerging. Food pattern modeling has been used by previous DGACs, and it was found to be very useful in elucidating food grouping nutrient profiles, for example. In the future such modeling will help to make much more sense out of the complex system of exposure that is diet, which influences health. Moreover, systems approaches (now in their infancy in the nutrition field) will help us to more clearly define the roles and limitations of diet in reducing chronic disease risk. A concentrated effort will be needed to help the *DGA* achieve its promise, particularly as its scope becomes broadened to include all Americans—not just healthy Americans—as well as children under 24 months and pregnant women.

As chair of the committee, I would like to thank members of the committee for their time, effort, and willingness to engage in these discussions. This National Academies Committee to Review the Process to Update the *Dietary Guidelines for Americans* wishes to sincerely thank the many experts who helped us with this report by giving presentations, writing comments, and reviewing our drafts. The review of this report was done by individuals chosen for their diverse perspectives as well as technical expertise, and we have greatly appreciated their input. The committee hopes actions that follow the release of this report will lead to a more transparent process, resulting in more trustworthy *DGA*.

Robert M. Russell, *Chair*
Committee to Review the Process to Update the
Dietary Guidelines for Americans

Acknowledgments

The committee and staff would like to thank those who made presentations and statements at the public workshop held on January 10, 2017, in Washington, DC, as well as those who submitted written comments for consideration during that meeting:

Angela Amico, Center for Science in the Public Interest, on behalf of Lorrene Ritchie, University of California Nutrition Policy Institute
Tejas Bhatt, Institute of Food Technologists
Darlena Birch, National Women, Infants, and Children Association
Patricia Britten, Center for Nutrition Policy and Promotion, U.S. Department of Agriculture (retired)
Cara Brumfield, 1,000 Days
Robert Burns, Grocery Manufacturers Association
Stephanie Chang, Agency for Healthcare Research and Quality
Jeannette Crenshaw, United States Breastfeeding Committee
Janet de Jesus, National Institutes of Health
Becky Domokos-Bays, Supervisor of School Nutrition, Loudoun County, VA
Eve Essery-Stoody, U.S. Department of Agriculture
Emma Gregory, American Frozen Food Institute
Colette Heimowitz, Atkins Nutritionals, Inc.
Guy Johnson, McCormick Science Institute
Casey Keller, Global Wrigley
Mark Kennedy, Physicians Committee for Responsible Medicine

Clara Lau, National Cattlemen's Beef Association
Susan Levin, Physicians Committee for Responsible Medicine
Sean Lucan, Albert Einstein College of Medicine
Richard Lucas, Food and Nutrition Service, U.S. Department of Agriculture
Patricia Mabry, Indiana University
David Meltzer, University of Chicago
Shawna Mercer, Centers for Disease Control and Prevention
Barbara Millen, Chair, 2015 Dietary Guidelines Advisory Committee
Suzanne Murphy, University of Hawaii Cancer Center
Julie Obbagy, U.S. Department of Agriculture
Jim O'Hara, Center for Science in the Public Interest
Sarah Ohlhorst, American Society for Nutrition
Mary Pat Raimondi, Academy of Nutrition and Dietetics
Tia Rains, Egg Nutrition Center
Kathleen Rasmussen, Cornell University
Pauline Sakamoto, Human Milk Banking Association of North America
Lee Sanders, American Bakers Association
Holger Schunemann, McMaster University
Kristen Strader, Public Citizen
Cathie Woteki, U.S. Department of Agriculture
Joan Younger, American Academy of Pediatrics Section on Breastfeeding
Tracey Ziener, Wrigley

We would like to thank those who provided written public comment to the committee. We would also like to recognize the General Services Administration for its helpful background information. In addition, there are many National Academies of Sciences, Engineering, and Medicine staff members who helped throughout the study process. The staff would like to thank Sylara Marie Cruz, Faye Hillman, Sarah Kelley, Tina Ritter, and Julie Wiltshire. Finally, we would like to thank and recognize the U.S. Department of Agriculture for sponsoring this study and for its helpful background information.

Contents

APPENDIXES

Acronyms and Abbreviations

AHA	American Heart Association
AHRQ EPC	Agency for Healthcare Research and Quality Evidence-based Practice Centers Program
AI	adequate intake
AMDR	Acceptable Macronutrient Distribution Range
AMSTAR	A Measurement Tool to Assess Systematic Reviews
ARS	U.S. Department of Agriculture Agricultural Research Service
ARS NND	Agricultural Research Service National Nutrient Database for Standard Reference
B–24	children from birth to 24 months
CDC	Centers for Disease Control and Prevention
COI	conflict of interest
CSFII	Continuing Survey of Food Intakes by Individuals
DASH	Dietary Approaches to Stop Hypertension
DAT	data analysis team
DGA	*Dietary Guidelines for Americans*
DGAC	Dietary Guidelines Advisory Committee
DGPCG	Dietary Guidelines Planning and Continuity Group
DGSAC	Dietary Guidelines Scientific Advisory Committee
DRI	Dietary Reference Intake

EAR	Estimated Average Requirement
EER	Estimated Energy Requirement
FDA	U.S. Food and Drug Administration
FTE	full-time equivalent
HHS	U.S. Department of Health and Human Services
IOM	Institute of Medicine
NEL	Nutrition Evidence Library
NEL BAT	Nutrition Evidence Library Bias Assessment Tool
NHANES	National Health and Nutrition Examination Survey
NHIS	National Health Interview Survey
NIH	National Institutes of Health
P/B–24	pregnant women and children from birth to 24 months
PICO	population, intervention/exposure, comparator, and outcome of interest
RDA	Recommended Dietary Allowance
SEER	National Cancer Institute's Surveillance, Epidemiology, and End Results
TEP	technical expert panel
UL	Tolerable Upper Intake Level
USDA	U.S. Department of Agriculture
WHO	World Health Organization
WIC	Special Supplemental Nutrition Program for Women, Infants, and Children
WWEIA	What We Eat in America

Summary[1]

This is the second and final report to examine and recommend ways to improve the process used to update the *Dietary Guidelines for Americans* (*DGA*). What foods should Americans eat to promote their health, and in what amounts? What is the scientific evidence that supports specific recommendations for dietary intake to reduce the risk of multifactorial chronic disease? These questions are critically important because dietary intake has been recognized to have a role as a key determinant of health. Some relationships between diet and health, such as under- or over-consumption of certain micronutrients, have been well established. For example, an individual whose diet lacks iron can develop iron-deficiency anemia. However, through years of scientific investigation in nutrition and health, an understanding that there are complex relationships between dietary intake and the risk of developing multifactorial chronic disease has been developing. Poor dietary habits have been associated with the increased prevalence of chronic diseases such as type 2 diabetes and cardiovascular disease in the United States. Likewise, poor-quality diets that result in energy imbalance can increase the risk of obesity. Diet is a multidimensional exposure, and metabolic responses to diet are varied. While the presence of a relationship between dietary habits and multifactorial chronic disease can be identified, the precise relationship between dietary patterns and health is complex, involving dynamic inter-

[1] This summary does not include references. Citations for the findings presented in the summary appear in subsequent chapters of the report.

actions among physical, social, behavioral, genetic, environmental, and other determinants of health. Because of this complexity, the responses to the questions of what Americans should eat and the supporting scientific evidence are not always simple ones.

As the primary federal source of consistent, evidence-based information on dietary practices for optimal nutrition, the *DGA* have the promise to empower Americans to make informed decisions about what and how much they eat to improve health and reduce the risk of chronic disease. In addition, the *DGA* serve as the basis for the types and composition of food provided in government food programs such as the National School Lunch Program and the Special Supplemental Nutrition Program for Women, Infants, and Children. Additionally, the *DGA* can be used as a basis for the development of more healthful products by food manufacturers. The individual and population uses of the *DGA* have the combined potential to improve population health. Unfortunately, most Americans do not consume a diet fully consistent with the *DGA*.

The adoption and widespread translation of the *DGA* require that they be universally viewed as valid, evidence-based, and free of bias and conflicts of interest to the extent possible. This has not routinely been the case. The *DGA* have been challenged, with critics questioning the validity of the evidence assessments. This has raised concerns in Congress about the trustworthiness of the *DGA*. This report recommends changes to the *DGA* process to reduce and manage sources of bias and conflicts of interest, improve timely opportunities for engagement by all interested parties, enhance transparency, and strengthen the science base of the process.

To help Americans make healthful food choices, the U.S. Department of Agriculture (USDA) and the U.S. Department of Health and Human Services (HHS) are mandated by Congress in the National Nutrition Monitoring and Related Research Act of 1990 to jointly review and author the guidelines every 5 years through a multistep process to reflect "the preponderance of the scientific and medical knowledge which is current at the time the report is prepared." The process to create the guidelines is not simple and has been modified as the science has evolved. In previous editions of the *DGA*, the process has begun with an assessment of relevant scientific data by a federal advisory committee selected and convened by USDA and HHS (see Figure S-1). This panel of nationally recognized experts, known as the Dietary Guidelines Advisory Committee (DGAC), independently evaluates the scientific evidence and makes recommendations to the departments about how the previous *DGA* could be revised. The conclusions of the DGAC are submitted to the secretaries of USDA and HHS in the form of a scientific report and are only advisory; they do not constitute draft policy. The *DGAC Scientific Report* serves as the scientific basis for the next edition of the *DGA*.

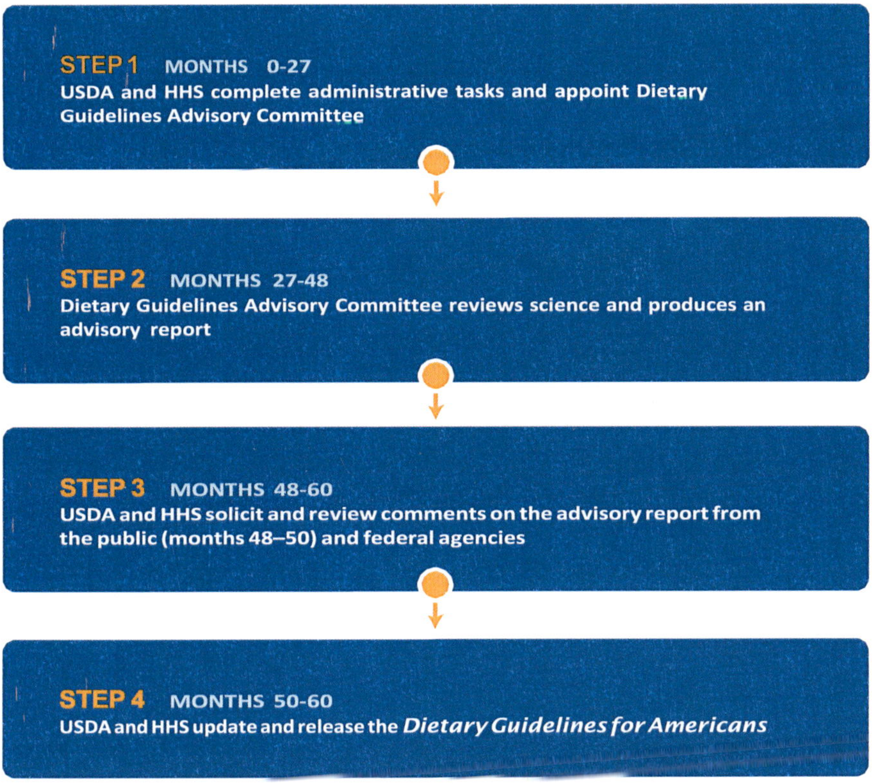
STEP 1 MONTHS 0-27
USDA and HHS complete administrative tasks and appoint Dietary Guidelines Advisory Committee
STEP 2 MONTHS 27-48
Dietary Guidelines Advisory Committee reviews science and produces an advisory report
STEP 3 MONTHS 48-60
USDA and HHS solicit and review comments on the advisory report from the public (months 48–50) and federal agencies
STEP 4 MONTHS 50-60
USDA and HHS update and release the *Dietary Guidelines for Americans*

FIGURE S-1 Primary steps for updating the *DGA*.
NOTES: Timeline based on the *2015–2020 DGA*. "Month" values indicate the approximate number of months after release of the previous edition of the *DGA*. HHS = U.S. Department of Health and Human Services; USDA = U.S. Department of Agriculture.

CHARGE TO THE NATIONAL ACADEMIES OF SCIENCES, ENGINEERING, AND MEDICINE

More than 29,000 public comments were submitted in response to the *Scientific Report of the 2015 DGAC* both in support of and against the conclusions made. The predominant topic addressed in the public comments was added sugars, with suggestions ranging from overall limitations to "a focus on total calories and portion sizes." The 2015 DGAC's inclusion of sustainability concerns was also controversial. In response to these criticisms, Congress mandated that the National Academies of Sciences, Engineering, and Medicine (the National Academies) evaluate the entire process used to develop the *DGA*. Specifically, the Consolidated Appropriations Act, 2016, calls for a review of the following (see Box 1-3 for the full Statement of Task):

1. How the advisory committee selection process can be improved to provide more transparency, eliminate bias, and include committee members with a range of viewpoints;
2. How the Nutrition Evidence Library (NEL) is compiled and utilized, including whether NEL reviews and other systematic reviews and data analysis are conducted according to rigorous and objective scientific standards;
3. How systematic reviews are conducted on long-standing *DGA* recommendations, including whether scientific studies are included from scientists with a range of viewpoints; and
4. How the *DGA* can better prevent chronic disease, ensure nutritional sufficiency for all Americans, and accommodate a range of individual factors, including age, gender, and metabolic health.

The National Academies appointed 14 members to the Committee to Review the Process to Update the *Dietary Guidelines for Americans*. Specifically, the task is to assess the *process* used to develop the guidelines and not evaluate the substance or use of the guidelines. A response to question 1, "How the advisory committee selection process can be improved to provide more transparency, eliminate bias, and include committee members with a range of viewpoints?" was published for the purpose of informing the 2020 cycle in a first short report, *Optimizing the Process for Establishing the* Dietary Guidelines for Americans: *The Selection Process*. This second report responds to the remaining questions through a comprehensive review of the process to update the *DGA*.

FINDINGS AND CONCLUSIONS

Upon evaluating the current process used to update the *DGA*, this National Academies committee found that the process has become more evidence-based over its more than 30-year history as demonstrated by the formal integration of food pattern modeling and the ability to conduct original systematic reviews. However, the entire process has not been comprehensively reconsidered in a manner that effectively allows it to adapt to changes in food diversity and chronic disease prevalences, while also protecting the integrity of the process. Specific to the process, the findings and conclusions of this National Academies committee are as follows:

1. The purpose and target audiences of the *DGA* have not been consistently interpreted, giving rise to confusion.
2. The juxtaposition of the 5-year *DGA* cycle and the 2-year DGAC term imposed by the National Nutrition Monitoring and Related Research Act and the Federal Advisory Committee Act constrain the overall system (e.g., time to complete tasks, structure). Additionally, because the DGAC has conducted all tasks of the scientific review, opportunities for a truly deliberative process with the nutrition community, technical experts, and the public are limited.
3. Transparency of the overall process to update the *DGA* needs improvement. For example, what standards are used to translate the evidence into recommendations and why the final *DGA* deviate from the conclusions of the *DGAC Scientific Report* have not been clearly explained. The current process also lacks a diversity of viewpoints and mechanisms to be responsive to topics of high public interest.
4. The methodological approaches to evaluating the scientific evidence require increased rigor to better meet current standards of practice. The *2010* and *2015–2020 DGA* were based on four types of analyses: (1) original systematic reviews; (2) existing systematic reviews, meta-analyses, and reports; (3) food pattern modeling;[2] and (4) descriptive data analyses. The basic steps for conducting each analysis are generally reasonable; however, there are many ways in which the analyses need to be strengthened. For example, the NEL systematic review protocol lacks a clear separation of functions between the primary actors: the DGAC and the NEL. Additionally, the procedure by which the NEL protocol is updated to take into account advances in systematic review methods is not clear.
5. Several aspects of the current approach to the scientific review would benefit from revision. First, the long duration between systematic reviews on a topic under the current system often does not keep pace with the emerging science; thus, ongoing surveillance of the literature needs to be instituted. Second, food pattern modeling is generally well designed for the questions it is intended to answer related to the average American diet, but its applicability to those who follow a different consumption pattern has been limited. Lastly, the processes to identify nutrients

[2] Food pattern modeling refers to analyses that incorporate various data inputs, constraints, goals, and assumptions to assess the nutrient content of various possible eating patterns based on typical choices within food groups.

of concern would benefit from further standardization.[3] Further integration of biochemical and health-related data in a systematic and consistent manner in the classification of nutrients of public health concern is also important.

6. There is a lack of mechanistic data to support incorporation of newly identified diet-related health conditions in future *DGA*. Analytic frameworks also are needed to guide topic selection and evidence review toward the synthesis and interpretation of analyses.

Collectively, these findings and conclusions suggest the integrity of the *DGA* is compromised and the ability to develop a full body of evidence on a continuous basis over time is limited. The process to update the *DGA* should be comprehensively redesigned to allow it to adapt to changes in needs, evidence, and strategic priorities.

VALUES OF AN EFFECTIVE PROCESS TO UPDATE THE *DGA*

Based on the key findings, this National Academies committee identified five values to improve the integrity of a process to develop credible and trustworthy guidelines:

1. Enhance transparency.
2. Promote diversity of expertise and experience.
3. Support a deliberative process.
4. Manage biases and conflicts of interest.
5. Adopt state-of-the-art processes and methods.

The process to update the *DGA* is also time- and resource-intensive. To the extent possible, a more efficient use of resources ought to be considered to minimize duplication of efforts and simplify the *DGA* without endangering its integrity. Implementing these values in the process to update the *DGA* will require that significant changes be made, necessitating a commitment from both USDA and HHS to ultimately achieve sustained performance.

Transparency is vital to engendering trust in the process, and it provides assurance that decisions were made free of undue influences. Each step of the process needs to be documented and updated, and such documentation needs to be readily available to the public. Opportuni-

[3] Nutrients of concern are nutrients that may be a substantial public health concern and are determined by evaluating the prevalence of nutrient inadequacies and excesses in the U.S. population and select population groups.

ties for meaningful public participation and engagement will need to be enhanced. However, in the steps of the process where public participation would be inappropriate, such as decision making, it will be critical to explain why key decisions were made.

Trustworthiness of the process can also be enhanced by increasing opportunities for stakeholder participation, particularly by involving a broad range of expertise and experience, at appropriate times throughout the process by which the *DGA* are produced. Encouraging participation from stakeholders who represent a wide variety of perspectives—including the public, academia and researchers, advocacy groups, professional organizations, the food sector, and federal agencies—is critical to fostering diversity. All stakeholders could provide input into the process; however, only experts as appointed by the secretaries of USDA and HHS meeting bias and conflict-of-interest criteria ought to be involved in decision-making processes.

A more deliberative approach can help a process adapt to dynamic shifts in the system in which it operates. Characteristics of a deliberative process include supporting adaptability, continuity, and continuous learning. The breadth and content of each required report could vary such that *not all topics* may require a detailed review every 5 years; only those topics with enough new data to generate a full review would be considered for in-depth evaluation in the next *DGA* cycle. Second, to facilitate a deliberative process, the *DGA* cycles need to be considered as a continuous activity to foster learning across cycles. Continuity also allows a strategic approach be developed to accomplish the goals and vision of the *DGA*. Third, the *DGA* process itself needs to continuously evolve and improve dynamically in response to advances in science.

An effective process also needs to ensure independence in decision making. The process redesign will need to align the roles and responsibilities at each step of the process with appropriate experts involved in decision making. Actual or perceived conflicts of interest—both financial and nonfinancial—will need to be eliminated to the extent possible or their effects minimized and managed.

Finally, scientific rigor needs to be maximized. The process by which the science is evaluated can be strengthened by (1) using validated, standardized processes and methods; and (2) using the most up-to-date data. Processes and actions ought to be based on the best available evidence, requiring that the types of analysis used be continuously improved and advanced.

BROADENING THE SCOPE OF THE *DGA*

A fundamental shift is required such that future *DGA* focus on the general public across the entire life span, and not just healthy Americans ages 2 years and older. Given the range of metabolic health and the prevalence of chronic diseases in the population, as well as the importance of nutrition to pregnant women and children from birth to 24 months,[4] it is essential that the *DGA* be developed for all Americans whose health could benefit by improving diet. Numerous organizations have developed or endorsed population- or disease-specific guidelines. However, the *DGA* are not designed to adjudicate among them. Confusion regarding which guidelines to follow could be reduced by identifying areas of consistency among guidelines developed in a manner in line with the methods used in the *DGA*.

PROCESS REDESIGN

This National Academies committee concluded that process redesign for updating the *DGA* can improve transparency, promote diversity of expertise and experience, support a deliberative process, promote independence in decision making, and strengthen scientific rigor. If successfully implemented, these modifications collectively have the potential to help improve the credibility of the *DGA* and trustworthiness of the process. Redesign can also improve the agility of the process and promote continuity of focus in key areas. Redesign that allows for the on-demand acquisition of many resources and an expanded set of multidisciplinary experts can improve the efficiency of the process. Redesign can also address needs for improved continuity between *DGA* cycles in areas such as real-time monitoring and curation of new evidence, with a consistent focus on strategic objectives. A more agile, efficient, and effective process can improve the relevance and usefulness of the *DGA*, which may improve adherence to the guidelines.

This National Academies committee considers that the 5-year cycle time can be leveraged more effectively by redistributing the tasks of the DGAC (the aforementioned group of experts appointed to assess the science) to other entities. While separation of tasks adds additional components and potentially cost to the overall process, more targeted expertise can be dedicated to completing a specific task, resulting in higher-quality inputs into the synthesis of evidence, and more time for deliberations, stakeholder engagement, and transparency-related activities. This pro-

[4] The Agricultural Act of 2014 mandates that pregnant women and children from birth to 24 months be included in the *2020–2025 DGA*.

posed process redesign model also permits much of the context setting and evidence development to be accomplished early on in the process.

> **Recommendation 1. The secretaries of the U.S. Department of Agriculture (USDA) and the U.S. Department of Health and Human Services (HHS) should redesign the *Dietary Guidelines for Americans* (*DGA*) process to prioritize topics to be reviewed in each *DGA* cycle, and redistribute the current functions of the Dietary Guidelines Advisory Committee to three separate groups:**
>
> **a. Dietary Guidelines Planning and Continuity Group to monitor and curate evidence generation, to identify and prioritize topics for inclusion in the *DGA*, and to provide strategic planning support across *DGA* cycles;**
>
> **b. Technical expert panels to provide content and methodological consultation during evaluation of the evidence; and**
>
> **c. Dietary Guidelines Scientific Advisory Committee to interpret the scientific evidence and draw conclusions.**

The redesign incorporates continuity across 5-year cycles, with some activities spanning across *DGA* cycles (see Figure S-2). A Dietary Guidelines Planning and Continuity Group (DGPCG) identifies topics and questions for review, as well as provides help with strategic planning. Subcommittees would be convened as needed to address specific topic areas. The redesign also creates an additional framework that would support the scientific needs of the process: technical expert panels (TEPs). The synthesis and interpretation of evidence, as well as development of conclusions, would be the primary focus of a Dietary Guidelines Scientific Advisory Committee (DGSAC). The secretaries of USDA and HHS would oversee the entire process.

The DGPCG is envisioned as a group of federal staff and nonfederal experts convened to perform the following three functions:

1. Provide the secretaries of USDA and HHS with planning support that assures alignment with long-term strategic objectives spanning multiple *DGA* cycles.
2. Identify and prioritize topics for the DGSAC to evaluate in subsequent *DGA* cycles.
3. Oversee monitoring and surveillance for new evidence.

These functions are consistent with the conclusion that not all topics need to be fully reevaluated every 5 years. Strategic planning is needed

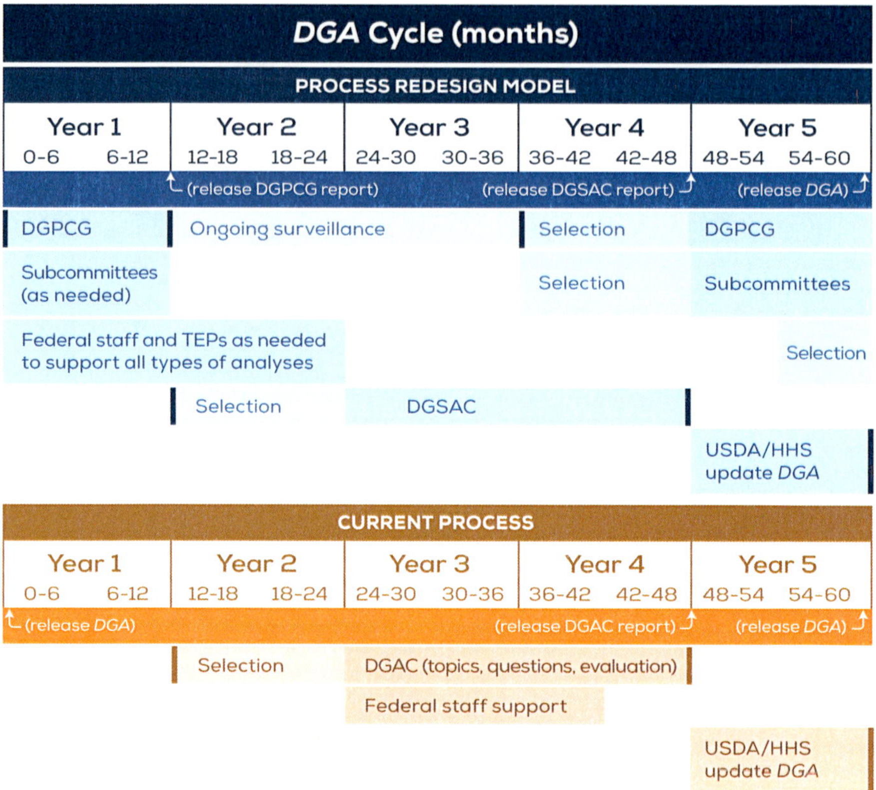

FIGURE S-2 Proposed timeline for future *DGA* cycles.
NOTES: Dark bars indicate opportunities for public comment and explanation of key decisions made. Darker shaded boxes indicate most active periods, while lighter shaded boxes denote potential times of less active engagement as needed. "Selection" refers to the selection of members for the respective groups. "Federal staff" includes those providing technical support such as the Nutrition Evidence Library staff and those conducting food pattern modeling and descriptive data analyses. *DGA* = *Dietary Guidelines for Americans*; DGAC = Dietary Guidelines Advisory Committee; DGPCG = Dietary Guidelines Planning and Continuity Group; DGSAC = Dietary Guidelines Scientific Advisory Committee; HHS = U.S. Department of Health and Human Services; TEP = technical expert panel; USDA = U.S. Department of Agriculture.

across *DGA* cycles. With respect to identifying and prioritizing topics, the DGPCG would be responsible for disclosing in a brief report the criteria and logic for the list of topics and associated research questions recommended. The DGPCG would also help oversee activities to monitor the scientific and public health literature to determine when enough new evidence has been developed on a specific topic, or when a topic is of high enough public interest, to warrant review for potential inclusion in a future *DGA* cycle. Functions 1 and 3 require that the DGPCG not be time limited and that it operate across *DGA* cycles. It is likely that additional expertise will be needed during the deliberations of the DGPCG. For example, fully vetting topic considerations may require expertise not covered by DGPCG members. The DGPCG could seek supplemental expertise in a number of ways including commissioned papers, invited speakers, consultants, advisors, roundtables, or subcommittees, depending on the breadth and complexity of the topic. A good model to consider for identifying questions for topics with broad subject matter is the project to expand the *DGA* to include women who are pregnant and children from birth to 24 months. That project engaged with a broad number of stakeholders with specialized expertise to identify and develop topics and questions for systematic reviews, while separating the topic identification process from the evidence evaluation.

TEPs, inclusive of nonfederal and federal experts in the domains of relevant methodologies with a diversity of scientific viewpoints, are proposed by this National Academies committee as a mechanism to supplement the technical insights in the beginning stages of any type of analysis. The number of such TEPs will vary based on needs during each *DGA* cycle.

In the process redesign model, the DGSAC is charged with developing evidence-based conclusions for USDA and HHS to consider in the next *DGA* update. Specifically, the DGSAC would be charged with integrating all data inputs such as systematic reviews, food pattern modeling, and descriptive data analyses in order to develop its conclusions regarding diet and its relationship to health. The DGSAC will need to determine a priori standards for evidence it will consider. As needed, the DGSAC would also be able to identify and request a limited number of new analyses. The DGSAC would deliver a scientific report that would serve as the scientific foundation for the *DGA Policy Report*. The DGSAC would also be charged with identifying topics where more evidence is needed, and suggesting those topics for future *DGA* cycles. Members of the DGSAC would include subject matter experts, as well as experts in the methods being considered for use in that particular *DGA* cycle (e.g., systematic reviews, food pattern modeling). Collectively, the experts involved with the DGPCG, TEPs, and DGSAC would represent a wide range of expertise and experience.

The structure of the process redesign model allows each group to focus on a major task of the proposed process: topic identification, selection, and prioritization; data collection and evaluation; data synthesis, interpretation, and integration; and the update of the *DGA*. Because the goals of topic identification, selection, and prioritization are different, it is this National Academies committee's opinion that specific criteria need to be defined for each stage, and that the public ought to participate in topic nomination. As soon as the DGPCG prioritizes topics for a particular *DGA* cycle and the secretaries of USDA and HHS affirm the list, the next task of collecting and evaluating data would begin. Teams of federal methodologists would work with TEPs to begin conducting systematic reviews, food pattern modeling, and descriptive data analyses (e.g., NEL staff, nutritional epidemiologists, respectively), with the goal of having final results available for the DGSAC when it first convenes. The DGSAC would then independently evaluate the evidence and develop conclusions, consulting with appropriate methodologists as needed to understand the evidence.

The federal writing team—the group that updates the *DGA* based on the scientific report—needs to adhere to explicit and transparent standards for developing evidence-based guidelines and recommendations. These standards ought to be incorporated into the *DGA* process and updated to align with best practices in the field. To enhance the integrity of the process, every effort needs to be made to ensure that the *DGA Policy Report* is transparent about what decisions were made about the DGSAC's conclusions, and the secretaries should explain why any deviations exist.

Recommendation 2. The secretaries of USDA and HHS should provide the public with a clear explanation when the *DGA* omit or accept only parts of conclusions from the scientific report.

This National Academies committee envisions the DGSAC as a federal advisory committee and the TEPs as ad hoc groups. Three options were considered for establishing the DGPCG: a federal advisory committee, a federal group, and a nongovernmental organization. Weighing the advantages and disadvantages reveals no perfect option. Establishing the DGPCG as a federal advisory committee ensures some mechanisms for objectivity and transparency but adds layers of complexity. A federal group would likely be the easiest to implement; however, it may not be viewed as independent. Although a nongovernmental organization could ensure transparency, it depends on identification of an influential, nonpartisan organization. This National Academies committee believes establishing the DGPCG as a federal advisory committee to be the most likely option to yield a trustworthy, dependable evaluation of the science. Regardless of which option is selected, the redesign will need to include experts with a diversity of scientific viewpoints.

STRENGTHENING ANALYSES AND ADVANCING METHODS USED

The *DGA* have to be based on the highest standards of scientific data and analyses to reach the most robust recommendations. The *DGA* require multiple sources of evidence to address the breadth of its scope. Data will need to come from varying study designs, such as randomized trials and observational studies. These aggregate data, analyzed with the most current methodology, provide complementary evidence to answer different inferential questions and inform various parts of the evidence base. Properly evaluating and calibrating results from a variety of data sources and methodological approaches is critical to understanding and interpreting the body of evidence to arrive at appropriate conclusions, as all study designs have innate limitations and can be susceptible to different types of bias. The dual challenge faced in developing the *DGAC Scientific Report*, and subsequently the *DGA* recommendations, is to properly assess the quality and interpret the results of studies available, and to use them appropriately in drawing conclusions about the body of evidence. Taking the limitations of evidence sources into account is crucial for building guidelines that are based on the totality of scientific evidence. Strengthening the current analyses depends on using the best data and the most rigorous processes and methods available. Advancing the evidence underpinning the *DGA* will also require integrating newer methods that help better elucidate and represent the complex systems involved.

Strengthening the NEL process for conducting de novo systematic reviews and identifying appropriate existing systematic reviews will require a multipronged approach. Clearly delineating the roles of the DGSAC and the NEL staff, as well as incorporating formal peer review, would ensure appropriate methods are used and would minimize the risk of bias in conducting systematic reviews. It is also critical to incorporate the appropriate expertise at specific steps in the protocol.

Recommendation 3. The secretary of USDA should clearly separate the roles of USDA Nutrition Evidence Library (NEL) staff and the Dietary Guidelines Scientific Advisory Committee (DGSAC) such that

a. The NEL staff plan and conduct systematic reviews with input from technical expert panels, perform risk of bias assessment of individual studies, and assist the DGSAC as needed.

b. The NEL systematic reviews are externally peer reviewed prior to being made available for use by the DGSAC.

c. The DGSAC synthesizes and interprets the results of systematic reviews and draws conclusions about the entire body of evidence.

The NEL should also maintain state-of-the-art systematic review methods. By instituting ongoing training and collaboration, as well as a supportive methodological infrastructure to cultivate practitioners of systematic review with a nutrition focus, the NEL has the opportunity to become a leading evidence source for the nutrition community. One opportunity to review implementation of methods is to invite experts in systematic review methodology to periodically review the NEL process. The NEL can learn from other organizations in particularly challenging steps of systematic reviews, such as implementation of grading criteria and evaluation of evidence. Another opportunity for collaboration and alignment with best practices is in synthesizing and interpreting the body of evidence. These are subjective processes and require experience and expertise. Thus, standard and up-to-date approaches are necessary to account for the strengths and the limitations of included studies and to formulate high-quality, evidence-based conclusions.

Recommendation 4. The secretary of USDA should ensure all Nutrition Evidence Library (NEL) systematic reviews align with best practices by

a. Enabling ongoing training of the NEL staff,
b. Enabling engagement with and learning from external groups on the forefront of systematic review methods,
c. Inviting external systematic review experts to periodically evaluate the NEL's methods, and
d. Investing in technological infrastructure.

Using high-quality systematic reviews from the literature whenever possible maximizes limited time and resources, as well as reduces duplication of efforts. However, this will require ongoing surveillance of the literature to ensure systematic reviews are up to date while at the same time leveraging resources.

Diet constitutes an extremely complex system of exposure that is known to influence health, and modeling can help to make sense of that complex system. More advanced food pattern modeling can increase the ability of the *DGA* to account for the complex systems involved and the variabilities in food composition and consumption. Food pattern models will be most useful as methods are strengthened to adapt to new areas of science, a better appreciation of the systems involved is formed, more systems science methods become available, and technology becomes increasingly more sophisticated.

Recommendation 5. The secretaries of USDA and HHS should enhance food pattern modeling to better reflect the complex interactions involved, variability in intakes, and range of possible healthful diets.

The accuracy and efficiency of data analyses could be improved by standardizing and validating the processes used, both within and between *DGA* cycles to identify nutrients of concern. Standardization would lead to consistent development of quantitative thresholds of inadequacy or excess and the integration of other supportive evidence to identify a nutrient of concern. This consistency would facilitate comparisons of descriptive data analyses over time, benefiting practitioners, consumers, and the food sector.

Recommendation 6. The secretaries of USDA and HHS should standardize the methods and criteria for establishing nutrients of concern.

The questions asked by previous DGACs have been, by necessity, limited by the types of evidence, data, and methods available. Advancing the evidence base will require not only strengthening existing data and types of analyses but also including new sources of evidence.

A systems approach is recommended to account for and understand the interrelated factors at play in both population and individual health. The *DGA* can play a key role in advancing the understanding of the role of diet within the larger body of evidence on factors that affect health. Constructing systems maps can lead to new insights and advance knowledge of the pathways connecting diet and health. Systems thinking, when fully integrated into the *DGA* process and supported with systems mapping and modeling, has the potential to influence the *DGA* recommendations based on comprehensive knowledge of the relationships of interest between diet and health. Systems thinking can also inform the translation of the guidelines to maximize impact and identify relevant connections across stakeholders.

Recommendation 7. The secretaries of USDA and HHS should commission research and evaluate strategies to develop and implement systems approaches into the *DGA*. The selected strategies should then begin to be used to integrate systems mapping and modeling into the *DGA* process.

1

Introduction

Federal advice to the public on nutrition and diet is intended to reflect the state of the science and deliver the most reliable recommendations according to the best available evidence. This advice, presented in the *Dietary Guidelines for Americans* (*DGA*), underpins all federal nutrition policies and programs and is updated every 5 years. The process to create the guidelines is not a simple one, and it changes as the science evolves. Much has been accomplished to improve how the science is evaluated and translated into the *DGA*, such as the establishment of the Nutrition Evidence Library (NEL) to conduct evidence-based reviews. The target population for the *DGA* will also expand in the 2020–2025 edition to include recommendations for all Americans by including pregnant women and children from birth to 2 years.

Despite the many accomplishments, recent challenges to federal nutrition guidance prompted Congress to question the process by which food and nutrition guidance is developed (Conaway, 2015; Hartzler et al., 2015; U.S. Congress, House of Representatives, Committee on Agriculture, 2015). To address these questions, Congress mandated a review of the entire process used to develop the *DGA*.[1]

[1] Consolidated Appropriations Act, 2016. Public Law 114-113, 114th Cong. (December 18, 2015), 129 Stat. 2280–2281.

THE *DIETARY GUIDELINES FOR AMERICANS*

The *DGA* provide nutritional and dietary information to promote health and prevent disease (HHS/USDA, 2015). To help Americans make healthful food choices, the U.S. Department of Agriculture (USDA) and the U.S. Department of Health and Human Services (HHS) jointly review and update the guidelines every 5 years to reflect "the preponderance of the scientific and medical knowledge which is current at the time the report is prepared."[2] The process to develop the guidelines has evolved over time in an effort to develop gold-standard guidelines. The guidelines are formed through a multistep process developed by USDA and HHS. USDA and HHS receive input from a scientific advisory committee, other federal agencies, and the public (see Figure 1-1).

While the term *DGA* has been used generally to refer to the report and the specific guidelines, for the purpose of clarity, more specific terminology is used throughout this National Academies of Sciences, Engineering, and Medicine (the National Academies) report (see Box 1-1).

Since the first edition in 1980, the guidelines have served as the basis for federal nutrition policies and nutrition assistance programs, as well as nutrition education programs.[3] Box 1-2 provides examples of how the *DGA* are used at various levels of government.

Overview of the Process to Update the *DGA*

First, a charter is filed with Congress to establish a scientific advisory committee, known as the Dietary Guidelines Advisory Committee (DGAC). The advisory committee comprises nationally recognized experts responsible for independently evaluating the scientific evidence to inform revisions to the current policy or suggest new guidance. Its conclusions are submitted to the secretaries of USDA and HHS as the *Scientific Report of the Dietary Guidelines Advisory Committee*. The DGAC's report

[2] National Nutrition Monitoring and Related Research Act of 1990, Public Law 101-445, 101st Cong. (October 22, 1990), 7 U.S.C. 5341, 104 Stat. 1042–1044. The departments are required to act within the National Nutrition Monitoring and Related Research Act of 1990, Agricultural Act of 2014, Federal Advisory Committee Act of 1972, and the Consolidated Appropriations Act of 2001 (Data Quality Act) (USDA/HHS, 2016).

[3] Federal nutrition assistance and education programs include Child and Adult Care Food Program; Commodity Supplemental Food Program; Food Distribution Program on Indian Reservations; Fresh Fruit and Vegetable Program; National School Lunch Program; Nutrition Services Incentive Program; Nutrition Standards for School Meals; School Breakfast Program; Serving Up MyPlate; SNAP-Ed; Special Milk Program; Special Supplemental Nutrition Program for Women, Infants, and Children (WIC); Summer Food Service Program; Supplemental Nutrition Assistance Program; Team Nutrition; The Emergency Food Assistance Program; USDA Foods–School Resources; and WIC Works.

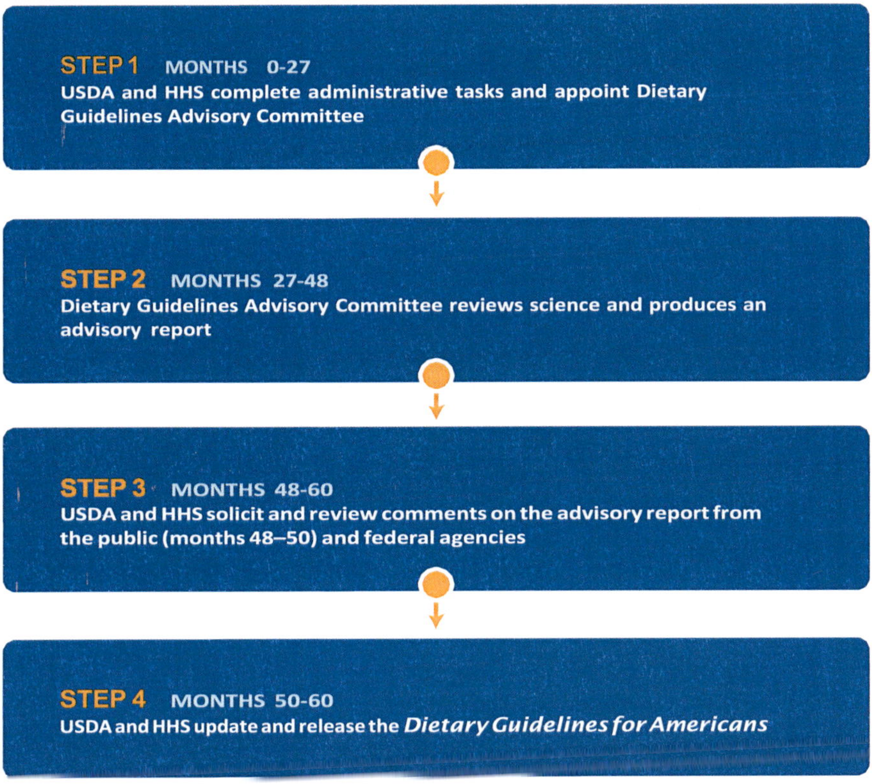
STEP 1 MONTHS 0-27
USDA and HHS complete administrative tasks and appoint Dietary Guidelines Advisory Committee
STEP 2 MONTHS 27-48
Dietary Guidelines Advisory Committee reviews science and produces an advisory report
STEP 3 MONTHS 48-60
USDA and HHS solicit and review comments on the advisory report from the public (months 48–50) and federal agencies
STEP 4 MONTHS 50-60
USDA and HHS update and release the Dietary Guidelines for Americans

FIGURE 1-1 Primary steps for updating the *DGA*.
NOTES: Timeline based on the *2015–2020 DGA*. "Month" values indicate the approximate number of months after release of the previous edition of the *DGA*. HHS = U.S. Department of Health and Human Services; USDA = U.S. Department of Agriculture.
SOURCE: Adapted from USDA, 2016b.

serves as the scientific basis for the *DGA*, but its conclusions are advisory in nature only; the scientific report does not constitute draft policy.

The secretaries then solicit comments on the *DGAC Scientific Report* from the public and other federal agencies. Next, a federal writing team—consisting of staff from USDA and HHS—collects, assesses, and reviews these comments as it develops the next edition of the *DGA Policy Report*. The draft *DGA Policy Report* undergoes a series of internal departmental reviews, including reviews by more than 100 subject-matter experts from the federal government, and revisions prior to approval by the secretaries. Finally, the *DGA Policy Report* is published publicly with the primary

BOX 1-1
Use of the Term *DGA* Throughout This National Academies Report

The term *DGA* has been broadly used in the nutrition community over time to refer to the *DGA* report itself, as well as the specific dietary guidelines that the *DGA* report describes. The *DGA* report integrates the science-based recommendations, which are based on a scientific report developed by the current Dietary Guidelines Advisory Committee (DGAC) into a form that can be used for policy development. Since 2005, the target audience for the *DGA* has been policy officials, nutritionists, and nutrition educators (USDA/HHS, 2016). For the purpose of clarity, more specific terminology is used throughout this National Academies report, although it is recognized that these terms may not be the operational terms used by the departments or the nutrition community.

- "DGA recommendations"[a] refers to the main messages from USDA and HHS—the most recent guidelines call for Americans to "follow a healthy eating pattern across the life span; focus on variety, nutrient density, and amount; limit calories from added sugars and saturated fats and reduce sodium intake; shift to healthier food and beverage choices; and support healthy eating patterns for all" and were accompanied by 13 supporting key recommendations (HHS/USDA, 2015).
- *DGA Policy Report* refers to the report released every 5 years by the secretaries of USDA and HHS in response to the National Nutrition Monitoring and Related Research Act. The 2015 version was titled the *Dietary Guidelines for Americans 2015–2020: Eighth Edition.* DGA recommendations and supporting evidence are first presented to the public in this document.
- *Dietary Guidelines Advisory Committee Scientific Report* denotes the document produced by the DGAC. The 2015 DGAC report was titled the *Scientific Report of the 2015 Dietary Guidelines Advisory Committee.* The conclusions from the scientific report serve as the scientific basis for the DGA Policy Report.
- "DGA" refers to all of the collective efforts and products to produce and disseminate the dietary guidelines.

[a] In some editions of the *DGA*, key recommendations were released in lieu of guidelines; others produced guidelines and/or key recommendations (see Appendix D). In this National Academies report, the term "*DGA* recommendations" will be used to refer to both guidelines and key recommendations.

audience being health professionals who then implement the guidelines through programs supported by federal, state, and local governments (see Appendix D for a list of the *DGA* recommendations since 1980).

BOX 1-2
Examples of Government Applications of the *Dietary Guidelines for Americans*

The key recommendations provided in the *Dietary Guidelines for Americans* (*DGA*) *Policy Report* are intended to be translated into action to help Americans consume healthful diets. One of the main functions of the guidelines is to provide food-based guidance for federal nutrition programs. These include but are not limited to the National School Lunch Program; the School Breakfast Program; the Special Supplemental Nutrition Program for Women, Infants, and Children (WIC); and the Child and Adult Care Food Program. Applications of the guidelines, however, include policies, nutrition programs (e.g., National School Lunch Program), education programs (e.g., SNAP-Ed, Choose MyPlate), and tools (e.g., Nutrition Facts labels) at the federal, state, and local levels.

Three specific examples are described below.

Aligning School Meal Standards with the DGA

As two nutrition programs administered by USDA, the National School Lunch Program and the School Breakfast Program must provide meals that are aligned with the *DGA*. The federal standards used for meal planning for these programs are assessed for adherence to the latest edition of the guidelines and, if needed, adjusted accordingly. The release of the *2010 DGA Policy Report*, for example, led to establishing vegetables as their own component, separate from fruits, in the National School Lunch Program. The Final Rule further specified that all vegetable subgroups defined in the *2010 DGA Policy Report* (dark green, red/orange, beans and peas [legumes], starchy, and other) must be provided over the course of a week.[a] Another change included in the National School Lunch Program and School Breakfast Program after the release of the *2010 DGA* was that only grains qualifying as "whole grain-rich" may be served.

Not all updates to the *DGA Policy Report* lead to substantial programmatic changes, and consideration is given to the feasibility of implementation. For example, compliance with the *2015–2020 DGA* recommendation of limiting added sugar to no more than 10 percent of calories was not readily implementable in the National School Lunch Program and School Breakfast Program with respect to competitive foods sold in the school setting. To put this recommendation into operation, the contribution of added sugars to total calories of each product would have to be known. This information is not currently listed on Nutrition Facts labels and is challenging to discern at present. Until added sugars are separately listed on Nutrition Facts labels, the standard for sugars will remain based on its contribution to the food products' total weight.

continued

BOX 1-2 Continued

Updating the Nutrition Facts Label

In May 2016, the U.S. Food and Drug Administration (FDA) announced changes to the Nutrition Facts labels intended to reflect current scientific evidence and help consumers make informed choices.[b] One revision is to list the amount of total sugars that come from added sugars. The FDA cites the revision as providing alignment with the *2015–2020 DGA Policy Report* key recommendation regarding added sugars (FDA, 2016). Another revision affects the percent daily values. The percent daily values show how much a serving of the food contributes to reference intake levels for a nutrient. The FDA updated the daily reference value for sodium, guided in part by the *2010 DGA Policy Report*; the key recommendation for sodium did not change with the *2015–2020 DGA Policy Report*.

Establishing Policies at the State Level

Although a primary role is to guide federal nutrition-related efforts, the *DGA Policy Report is* also used by policy makers and health professionals throughout the country. In 2009, Massachusetts became the first state to enact a statewide food procurement policy for state agencies.[c] The resulting nutrition standards developed by the Massachusetts Department of Health were based on the *2005 DGA Policy Report* (Massachusetts Executive Office of Health and Human Services, 2016) and have been reevaluated to ensure alignment with subsequent editions (Massachusetts Department of Public Health, 2012). Standards were set for each food group (e.g., milk provided to individuals 2 years and older must be low-fat or nonfat) and food preparation (e.g., elimination of deep fryers). Similarly, state agencies in Washington were required to begin implementing healthful food service guidelines as of July 1, 2014.[d] From this executive order came the *Healthy Nutrition Guidelines* (Washington State Department of Health, 2014), which follow the *2010 DGA Policy Report* and are provided for vending, meetings and events, cafeterias, and institutions.

---

[a] 7 C.F.R. § 210 and 220, 2012.

[b] 21 C.F.R. § 101, 2016.

[c] Massachusetts Executive Order 509, *Establishing Nutrition Standards for Food Purchased and Served by State Agencies* (2009).

[d] Washington Executive Order 13-06, *Improving the Health and Productivity of State Employees and Access to Healthy Foods in State Facilities* (2013).

Criticisms of the *2015–2020 DGA*

When the *Scientific Report of the 2015 Dietary Guidelines Advisory Committee* was released in February 2015, more than 29,000 written public comments were submitted. In contrast, approximately 2,000 comments were received in response to the *2010 DGAC Scientific Report* (U.S. Congress, House of Representatives, Committee on Agriculture, 2015). Of the statements received in 2015, approximately 21,000 submissions were form letters or petitions. Form letters were the major type of submission, comprising greater than 70 percent of all comments; 33 unique form letters were received. Approximately 187,000 signatures were received from 47 petitions. Critiques of the report itself and the process used—both in support of and against the conclusions—were raised for a wide range of topics. The predominant topic addressed was added sugars. Some remarks suggested a limitation on added sugars, while others promoted "a focus on total calories or portion sizes" (HHS, 2015). The issue of sustainability was also widely addressed and was the subject of a large majority of form letter submissions, most of which supported its inclusion. Many statements also referred to lean meat, largely questioning its lack of inclusion in the scientific report as part of a healthful diet, but others referenced concerns about cholesterol and saturated fat associated with meat consumption. Plant-based diets were another frequently identified topic, with comments both in favor of and against a shift to a more plant-based diet. A variety of other comments were received, such as suggestions to focus on a specific micronutrient or macronutrient, making the guidelines easier to apply, and specific critiques about the processes used by both the DGAC and the method it used to evaluate the science (HHS, 2015).

In part because of the large number of comments, Congress raised questions about the scope of the 2015 DGAC, stating that the DGAC did not have the expertise, evidence, or charter to comment on topics such as sustainable diets and tax policy (Conaway, 2015; Hartzler et al., 2015). Others raised questions regarding the evidence used and the comprehensiveness of the literature reviewed (Dabrowska, 2016; Heimowitz, 2016; Hentges, 2016; Mozzaffarian, 2016; Teicholz, 2015). Following an examination of these public comments, the House Committee on Agriculture held a hearing where the secretaries of USDA and HHS were asked to clarify, among other things, that the *DGAC Scientific Report* was based in science and that sustainability concerns were outside the scope of the DGAC. Congress also raised questions about the process to develop the *DGA*, asking whether the process could be trusted by the American people, and demanding that the *DGA* be developed in a transparent and objective manner (U.S. Congress, House of Representatives, Committee on Agriculture, 2015).

After the release of the *Dietary Guidelines for Americans 2015–2020: Eighth Edition* in January 2016, USDA invited 40 stakeholders to voice support or concern for the process of developing the *DGA*. Ten professional organizations were represented, as well as 18 members of industry and 12 individuals with various background and professional associations. A summary of the comments received related to the composition and the selection process of the DGAC can be found in this National Academies committee's first report (NASEM, 2017). Comments from the listening session were made both in favor of and against the current processes used to develop the *DGA Policy Report*. Frequently discussed topics included the processes used to create the *DGA Policy Report* and the *DGAC Scientific Report*, as well as how evidence was assessed for the scientific report. Also commonly mentioned was the timing of when research questions are developed, as well as the suggestion to provide more opportunities to comment on the questions for the DGAC to consider before it conducts its work. Commenters discussed the periodicity of the *DGA*, with some arguing for more frequent editions and others suggesting less frequent revisions.

Greater transparency into the process to translate the *DGAC Scientific Report* into the *DGA Policy Report* was also raised as a point for potential improvement. The potential conflict of interest USDA might have in managing and supporting the *DGA* given its role in supporting U.S. agriculture, as well as potential influence from Congress and the food sector, was also raised. Others suggested that USDA and HHS might be reluctant to make changes that would contradict previous guidelines. Statements were also presented regarding the literature review process—approximately half were positive—with others suggesting that the DGAC evaluate how it interprets and considers different study types. Many presenters also stated their support for the NEL process as being evidence-based, transparent, and held to rigorous scientific standards. Others critiqued the NEL, challenging its comprehensiveness, the DGAC's inconsistent use of the NEL, and lack of public access to the NEL's work throughout the DGAC process. Numerous suggestions were also made about measuring the effectiveness of the *DGA* and developing education programs to strengthen the public health impact of the *DGA*. Calls were also made to clarify the target audience and the scope of both the *DGA* and the DGAC (USDA, 2016a).

EVALUATION BY THE NATIONAL ACADEMIES OF SCIENCES, ENGINEERING, AND MEDICINE

In response to concerns raised about the process to produce the *2015–2020 DGA Policy Report*, Congress directed USDA to engage with the

National Academies to appoint a committee to conduct a comprehensive evaluation of the *processes* used to establish the *DGA* (see Box 1-3 for the Statement of Task).

Importantly, this National Academies committee is not evaluating the substance of the guidelines or their use; its charge is to *assess the process*. As such, the findings in this report should not be considered as judgments about the quality of prior *DGA* or DGAC reports. The questions in the Statement of Task are divided and addressed in two reports. This National Academies committee's first report responded to the first part of the task for the purpose of informing the 2020 cycle. That report recommends a number of ways to enhance transparency in the selection process for DGAC members, including identifying and managing biases and conflicts of interest (NASEM, 2017) (see Box 1-4).

The conclusions and recommendations contained herein respond to parts 2–4 in the Statement of Task. Although most of the evidence and analysis related to the first question was discussed in the first report, some related issues are relevant to the present report and therefore are included. For example, the Agricultural Act of 2014 requested that the *DGA* be expanded to include people across the life span, adding guidance for pregnant women and children from birth to 24 months. Because this expansion may significantly affect the *DGA*—and by extension the DGAC—it affects the considerations for how the DGAC is composed and is thus discussed in this report. As part of this overall, comprehensive review of the process to update the *DGA*, additional findings and recommendations about the selection process are made. Additionally, some of the questions relevant to the selection process, such as how specific priority areas are determined and how the DGAC's conclusions are considered in the *DGA Policy Report*, are also explored here.

Committee Methods

The National Academies appointed 14 members to the Committee to Review the Process to Update the *Dietary Guidelines for Americans* to respond to a congressional request.[4] For this second report—to assess the rigor of the NEL, how systematic reviews are conducted on long-standing *DGA* recommendations, and how the *DGA* can better prevent chronic disease and ensure nutritional sufficiency for all Americans—this National Academies committee met in person twice and convened in closed session three times via webinar. Its discussions also benefited from engaging with the public; one in-person public comment session was

---

[4] Consolidated Appropriations Act, 2016, Public Law 114-113, 114th Cong. (December 18, 2015), 129 Stat. 2280–2281.

BOX 1-3
Statement of Task

An ad hoc committee will undertake an 18-month study to review the entire process used to establish the Advisory Committee for the *Dietary Guidelines for Americans* (DGAC) and the subsequent development of the *DGA*, most recently revised pursuant to section 301 of the National Nutrition Monitoring and Related Research Act of 1990 (7 U.S.C. § 5341). The committee will review the current processes for each of the following:

1. How the advisory committee selection process can be improved to provide more transparency, eliminate bias, and include committee members with a range of viewpoints;
2. How the Nutrition Evidence Library (NEL) is compiled and utilized, including whether NEL reviews and other systematic reviews and data analysis are conducted according to rigorous and objective scientific standards;
3. How systematic reviews are conducted on long-standing *DGA* recommendations, including whether scientific studies are included from scientists with a range of viewpoints; and
4. How the *DGA* can better prevent chronic disease, ensure nutritional sufficiency for all Americans, and accommodate a range of individual factors, including age, gender, and metabolic health.

The committee will produce a short report that includes a review of question 1 and, as needed, recommendations based on existing best practices for selecting a scientific advisory committee to inform development of the *DGA*. A final report will be produced that includes the committee's review of questions 2–4 and, as needed, recommendations based on existing practices for:

- Conducting and/or including rigorous and objective nutrition systematic reviews and other data analyses to support the development of the *DGA*;
- Supporting an expanded life span approach, specifically dietary guidance for infants up to 24 months and pregnant women (per the Agricultural Act of 2014);
- Effectively applying the *DGA* to prevent diet-related chronic disease in the United States using existing implementation and evaluation frameworks; and
- Identifying the role of the *DGA* in coordinating with and supporting nutrition guidance for disease treatment (that may also address age, gender, metabolic health, and nutritional sufficiency) developed by other federal agencies.

The committee's recommendations will conform to the specifications of the National Nutrition Monitoring and Related Research Act, Federal Advisory Committee Act, Data Quality Act, and align with the current infrastructure, availability of resources, and collaborative relationships led by the USDA Center for Nutrition Policy and Promotion (study sponsor) and the HHS Office of Disease Prevention and Health Promotion. The committee will not conduct systematic reviews of nutrition science, nor evaluate the content or scientific justification of current or previous editions of the *DGA*.

BOX 1-4
Recommendations for Selecting DGAC Members from *Optimizing the Process to Update the Dietary Guidelines for Americans: The Selection Process*

Recommendation 1. The secretaries of USDA and HHS should employ an external third party to review and narrow the candidate pool to a list of primary and alternate nominees. Criteria against which nominees are screened should be developed by USDA and HHS for use by the third party.

Recommendation 2. The secretaries of USDA and HHS should make a list of provisional appointees open for public comment—including short biographies and any known conflicts—for a reasonable period of time prior to appointment.

Recommendation 3. The secretaries of USDA and HHS should disclose how provisional nominees' biases and conflicts of interest are identified and managed by:

a. Creating and publicly posting a policy and form to explicitly disclose financial and nonfinancial biases and conflicts;
b. Developing a management plan for addressing biases and conflicts for the panel as a whole and individuals, as needed;
c. Certifying that a federal ethics officer independently reviewed and judged the advisory committee's biases and conflicts of interest; and by
d. Documenting how conflicts of interest were managed in the Dietary Guidelines Advisory Committee report.

Recommendation 4. The secretaries of USDA and HHS should adopt a system for continuous process improvement to enhance outcomes and performance of the Dietary Guidelines Advisory Committee selection process.

held, where members of the public were invited to address the committee. Those who made a statement included representatives of industry, professional organizations, advocacy groups, and individuals (see Appendix B). Additionally, the committee solicited written input from the public about what it believed to be major challenges to implementing the *DGA* and the greatest opportunities for the *DGA* to better prevent chronic disease and ensure nutritional sufficiency. Statements and comments were received by this National Academies committee from industry representatives, professional organizations, and interested individuals. All statements were considered over the course of the committee's deliberations.

Organization of This Report

This report consists of two parts to facilitate understanding of this National Academies committee's vision and recommendations for an improved process to update the *DGA*, particularly for those readers who are already familiar with the details of the current process. Part I of this report, inclusive of Chapters 2, 3, and 4, presents this National Academies committee's ideas and recommendations for how the *DGA* can better serve the American public in response to the Statement of Task. It describes a brief overview of the process to develop the *DGA*, the main findings and conclusions from this National Academies committee's evaluation, and recommendations. Chapter 2 describes this National Academies committee's vision for the roles and purposes of the *DGA*. Chapter 3 suggests a proposed model for the *DGA*. Chapter 4 provides recommendations for enhancing the science underlying the *DGA*.

Part II describes the current process in greater detail and this National Academies committee's analysis of the process and its evaluation of the evidence. Part II provides the basis for the conclusions and recommendations discussed in Part I. Chapter 5 describes and evaluates the current process for developing the *DGA* and presents findings that serve as the basis for the suggestions and recommendations in Chapter 3. In Chapter 5, this National Academies committee found that (1) the purposes and audiences of the *DGA* have not been consistently interpreted over time, (2) the cycle time and complexity of tasks constrain the current DGAC process, and (3) the current process is not as transparent or participatory as it could be.

Chapter 6 examines the types of analyses used to update the *2015–2020 DGA* and provides assessments upon which recommendations are made in response to Statement of Task questions "How is the Nutrition Evidence Library compiled and utilized, including whether NEL reviews and other systematic reviews and data analysis are conducted according to rigorous and objective scientific standards?" and "How are systematic reviews conducted on long-standing *DGA* recommendations, including whether scientific studies are included from scientists with a range of viewpoints?" This chapter asserts that the types of analyses used to update the *2015–2020 DGA*—(1) original systematic reviews; (2) existing systematic reviews, meta-analyses, and reports; (3) food pattern modeling; and (4) descriptive data analyses—provide important inputs into the *DGA* process. This National Academies committee found that the NEL process for conducting original systematic reviews is thorough but has not been updated to reflect recent advances in systematic review methodology. Additionally, the roles of the DGAC and NEL staff have not been clearly delineated in the *DGA* process. Although food pattern modeling has been conducted according to appropriate methods, it has been limited by the food groupings, assumptions, and constraints inherent in the models. Finally, descriptive data analyses conform to current approaches, but the DGAC's analyses can be limited by the availability of current data.

Chapter 7 reviews how previous DGACs considered nutritional adequacy and chronic disease, and it builds the basis for responding to the Statement of Task question "How can the *DGA* better prevent chronic disease, ensure nutritional sufficiency for all Americans, and accommodate a range of individual factors, including age, gender, and metabolic health?" This National Academies committee found that the process by which nutrients of concern are identified has yet to be standardized across *DGA* cycles. DGACs have yet to use an analytical framework to guide topic selection, synthesis, and interpretation of the evidence on topics of the relationship of diet, health, and chronic disease.

REFERENCES

Conaway, M. 2015. The science in our diet. *U.S. News & World Report.* http://www.usnews.com/opinion/articles/2015/10/05/why-the-science-behind-the-dietary-guidelines-matters (accessed June 8, 2017).

Dabrowska, A. 2016. Dietary Guidelines for Americans: *Frequently asked questions.* Washington, DC: Congressional Research Service (R44360).

FDA (U.S. Food and Drug Administration). 2016. *Changes to the Nutrition Facts label.* http://www.fda.gov/Food/GuidanceRegulation/GuidanceDocumentsRegulatoryInformation/LabelingNutrition/ucm385663.htm (accessed August 15, 2017).

Hartzler, V., M. Conaway, J. Walorski, K. Noem, and D. Webster. 2015. *Letter from members of Congress to the Honorable Tom Vilsack, Secretary of Agriculture and the Honorable Sylvia Mathews Burwell, Secretary of Health and Human Services (March 31, 2015).* http://agriculture.house.gov/uploadedfiles/ag_dietaryguidelineslettertosecsvilsackburwell.pdf (accessed June 8, 2017).

Heimowitz, C. 2016 (unpublished). *Comments presented at USDA* Dietary Guidelines for Americans *listening sessions: Atkins Nutritionals.* Washington, DC, February 19, 2016.

Hentges, E. 2016 (unpublished). *Comments presented at USDA* Dietary Guidelines for Americans *listening sessions: International Life Sciences Institute.* Washington, DC, February 19, 2016.

HHS (U.S. Department of Health and Human Services). 2015. *Public comments on the* Scientific Report of the 2015 Dietary Guidelines Advisory Committee. https://health.gov/dietaryguidelines/dga2015/comments/advisory-report-summary.asp (accessed January 5, 2017).

HHS/USDA (U.S. Department of Agriculture). 2015. Dietary Guidelines for Americans *2015–2020: Eighth edition.* https://health.gov/dietaryguidelines/2015/guidelines (accessed July 18, 2017).

Massachusetts Department of Public Health. 2012. *Massachusetts State Agency Food Standards: Requirements and recommendations.* http://www.mass.gov/eohhs/docs/dph/mass-in-motion/eo509-state-agency-food-standards.pdf (accessed June 2, 2017).

Massachusetts Executive Office of Health and Human Services. 2016. *Tools and resources for implementation of Executive Order 509.* http://www.mass.gov/eohhs/gov/departments/dph/programs/community-health/mass-in-motion/about-mim/components/tools-and-resources-for-executive-order-509.html (accessed March 2, 2017).

Mozzaffarian, D. 2016 (unpublished). *Comments presented at USDA* Dietary Guidelines for Americans *listening sessions.* Washington, DC, February 19, 2016.

NASEM (National Academies of Sciences, Engineering, and Medicine). 2017. *Optimizing the process for establishing the* Dietary Guidelines for Americans: *The selection process.* Washington, DC: The National Academies Press.

Teicholz, N. 2015. The scientific report guiding the U.S. dietary guidelines: Is it scientific? *British Medical Journal* 351:h4962.

U.S. Congress, House of Representatives, Committee on Agriculture. 2015. *Hearing to review the development of the 2015* Dietary Guidelines for Americans. 114th Cong., 1st Sess. October 7.

USDA (U.S. Department of Agriculture). 2016a. Dietary Guidelines for Americans: *Listening sessions.* Washington, DC. https://www.cnpp.usda.gov/sites/default/files/dietary_guidelines_for_americans/ListeningSessionTranscript-2-19-16.pdf (accessed January 5, 2017).

USDA. 2016b (unpublished). *Understanding the committee's charge: A discussion with the sponsor*. Presentation to the Committee to Review the Process to Update the *Dietary Guidelines for Americans*, September 1.

USDA/HHS. 2016 (unpublished). Dietary Guidelines for Americans: *Process brief, sections 1–3*. Prepared for the Committee to Review the Process to Update the *Dietary Guidelines for Americans*.

Washington State Department of Health. 2014. *Healthy nutrition guidelines: Implementation guide for agencies, sites and vendors.* Healthy Communities (DOH 340-224).

Part I

This report is presented in two parts to facilitate understanding of this National Academies of Sciences, Engineering, and Medicine (the National Academies) committee's vision and recommendations for an improved process to update the *Dietary Guidelines for Americans* (*DGA*), particularly for those readers who are already familiar with the details of the current process. Part I presents this National Academies committee's judgments and recommendations to redesign the process to update the *DGA*. Part II provides a detailed description and evaluation of the process as it has been conducted in recent cycles. Part I consists of three chapters:

Chapter 2 provides this National Academies committee's vision for how the roles and purposes of the process to update the *DGA* could best support development of dietary guidelines that Americans can trust and follow.

Chapter 3 presents this National Academies committee's proposed process redesign model to help the *DGA* adapt to future changes in Americans' health.

Chapter 4 suggests how the evidence base for the *DGA* can be strengthened. This is a critical topic given that the *DGA* are required to be based on the preponderance of evidence.

This National Academies committee encourages readers who would like a more in-depth description of the *DGA* process to turn to Part II for a full accounting of the current process, inclusive of an evaluation and key findings.

2

Role and Purposes of the *Dietary Guidelines for Americans*: Evaluation and Findings

What foods should Americans eat to promote their health, and in what amounts should those foods be eaten? What is the scientific evidence that supports specific recommendations for dietary intake to reduce the risk of chronic disease? These questions are critically important because dietary intake has long been recognized to have a role as a key determinant of health (NRC, 1989; WHO, 2003). Some relationships between diet and health, such as under- or overconsumption of certain micronutrients, have been well established (IOM, 2001). For example, an individual whose diet lacks iron can develop iron-deficiency anemia (CDC, 1998; IOM, 2001; NRC, 1989). However, through years of scientific investigation in nutrition and health, an understanding has begun to develop that there are complex relationships between dietary intake and the risk of developing multifactorial chronic disease. Poor dietary habits have been associated with the increased prevalence of chronic diseases such as type 2 diabetes and cardiovascular disease in the United States. Likewise, poor-quality diets that result in an energy imbalance increase the risk of obesity (Erdrich et al., 2015; Hill et al., 2012; Stampfer et al., 2000). While the presence of a relationship between dietary habits and chronic disease can be identified, the precise relationship between dietary patterns and health is complex, involving dynamic interactions among physical, social, behavioral, genetic, environmental, and other determinants of health. Because of this complexity, the responses to the questions of what Americans should eat and the supporting scientific evidence are not always simple ones.

The *Dietary Guidelines for Americans* (*DGA*) is the one source that attempts to address these complicated issues. This National Academies of Sciences, Engineering, and Medicine (the National Academies) committee found it important to review the purposes and goals of the *DGA* to guide its deliberations about improving the current process, and presents those discussions and findings in this chapter. The chapter then articulates a set of values on which to base the committee's assessment of the *DGA* process. The chapter concludes by describing how the scope of the *DGA* could be broadened to include all Americans and not solely healthy Americans.

ROLE OF THE *DGA*

To help the public better understand what eating patterns may help to reduce risk of disease, the nutrition community has long sought to offer science-based advice on food and provide practical support for its uptake. Such advice was first introduced in the United States in the late 1890s, with the themes of variety, balance, and moderation. In the following decades, numerous food guides were published from a variety of sources; most were similar and identified a range of 7 to 10 food groups. In the 1950s, the U.S. Department of Agriculture (USDA) simplified its "Basic Seven" food groups to the "Basic Four," with the focus of being a "foundation diet"—a diet meeting the major portion of calories and nutrients needed, assuming that people would supplement their diets for the remainder of the calories and nutrients. In the 1970s, quantitative goals for intakes were set to make food guides more directive, but these efforts led to controversy in the field, as the diets needed to meet the goals differed greatly from the usual food patterns of average Americans. For example, in 1977, the U.S. Senate Select Committee on Nutrition and Human Needs recommended a set of dietary goals for Americans, calling for the public to expend as much or more energy (kcals) as it consumes and suggesting nutrient- and food-based targets. When those goals were publicly released, industry and the scientific community questioned whether the recommendations could be supported by available science. The general public was left confused, suggesting the need for a single, authoritative, and consistent set of advice on diet and health from the federal agencies. As a result, USDA and the U.S. Department of Health and Human Services (HHS) developed the *DGA*, which provide the general public with a single set of food-based advice (Welsh et al., 1992).[1]

[1] Per the National Nutrition Monitoring and Related Research Act of 1990, "At least every five years the Secretaries [of USDA and HHS] shall publish a report entitled '*Dietary Guidelines for Americans*.' Each report shall contain nutritional and dietary information and guidelines for the general public, and shall be promoted by each Federal agency in carrying out any Federal food, nutrition, or health program." Refer to Chapter 1, Box 1-1, for an explanation of how the term *DGA* is used throughout this National Academies report.

The *DGA* serve as the primary federal source of consistent, evidence-based general information on diet and nutrition. In this role, the *DGA* have the potential to empower Americans to make informed decisions about what and how much they eat to improve health and reduce the risk of chronic disease. To make the *DGA* attainable by the general population and subpopulations, the *DGA* have been designed to have an important role in federal food policies and programs. As the basis for the types and composition of food provided in government food programs, the *DGA* can be used as a basis for the development of and access to more healthful products by food manufacturers, supermarkets, restaurants and food service operations, and other segments of the food sector. The *DGA* have the potential to improve population health through enhanced adherence to the *DGA* recommendations by individuals and use of the *DGA* by the private and public sectors.

Despite this potential, less than 10 percent of Americans consume a diet fully consistent with the *DGA* (HHS/USDA, 2015; Krebs-Smith et al., 2010; Wilson et al., 2016). For example, many consume greater quantities of solid fats, added sugars, alcoholic beverages, and sodium than recommended. Why Americans fail to adhere to the *DGA* is uncertain. Multiple factors have been reported as causes for the lack of adoption of the *DGA*, including cost, taste, challenges with identifying practical strategies to bring about change, foods being unavailable, concern over the healthfulness of the guideline diets, and difficulty in making dietary change (Nicklas et al., 2013). Other causes may include the societal context driving eating patterns and people simply not being aware of the *DGA* recommendations. Confusion may exist as a result of the presence of numerous dietary guidelines or the perception that dietary guidelines are constantly evolving (e.g., recommendations on consumption of eggs have changed). Another potential reason for lack of adherence is that the public has "lost faith" in the *DGA* (U.S. Congress, House of Representatives, Committee on Agriculture, 2015). As raised by members of Congress, if the credibility of the guidelines is low or questionable, adherence to the guidelines is likely to be limited (U.S. Congress, House of Representatives, Committee on Agriculture, 2015).

Many of the potential reasons for lack of adherence to the *DGA* recommendations require review of the environmental and behavioral aspects of the food system and food consumption. However, questions related to the credibility and trustworthiness of the *DGA* recommendations can be addressed through review of the process by which they are developed. The adoption and widespread translation of the *DGA* require that they be universally viewed as valid, evidence based, and free of bias and conflicts of interest to the extent possible. This report provides recommended changes to the *DGA* process to reduce and manage sources of bias and conflicts of interest, improve timely opportunities for engagement by all interested parties, enhance transparency, and strengthen the science base of the process. Redesigning the process is an essential first step, but evaluation will also be needed to understand whether the public does in fact trust the process and, in the long-term, whether adherence to the *DGA* recommendations actually improves.

CLARIFYING THE PURPOSES OF THE *DGA*

The purpose and uses of the *DGA* have undergone subtle changes over their more than 30-year history (see Table 5-2 for a detailed evolution of the *DGA*).[2] This evolution has led to some confusion about what and for whom the *DGA* are intended. Indeed, upon review of materials related to the *2015–2020 DGA Policy Report*, more than 10 different statements can be found describing the purposes, goals, and intended audiences for the *DGA*. While many of these statements overlap, some are conflicting. Some of the confusion about the purposes and audiences of the *DGA* stems from the multiple outputs of the process used to derive the *DGA*, such as the *Dietary Guidelines Advisory Committee (DGAC) Scientific Report* and the *DGA Policy Report* (see Table 2-1).

The purposes of the *DGA* are also different from those of the Dietary Reference Intakes (DRI, described in more detail in Chapter 7 and Appendix E), which focus on recommendations for specific nutrients. The *DGA*, by contrast, are food-based recommendations. To promote clarity in understanding the purposes and audiences of the various products of the *DGA* process, this National Academies committee proposes specific functions and ultimate recipients for each product of the process used to update the *DGA* (see Table 2-1).

Some materials currently exist that appear to be consumer oriented but are developed for use by health professionals. Disseminations such as Choose MyPlate and SuperTracker are important tools. These Internet-based tools are useful, but they do not necessarily reach everyone that could benefit from following the *DGA*. This National Academies committee believes the *DGA* recommendations themselves need to be their own separate, consumer-oriented publication—similar to the brochure form that was produced prior to 2005—to clearly articulate the *DGA* recommendations to the general public. Both the proposed brochure and *DGA* disseminations will be important to communicate the guidelines to the public.

---

[2] Table 5-2 shows how the audience and format of the *DGA* have changed over time. Originally, the *DGA* were published as a brochure for consumers; the *DGA* are now lengthy reports written for policy officials, nutritionists, and nutrition educators.

TABLE 2-1 Delineating the Functions and Audiences of Products Related to the *DGA* Process

Product	Example	Audience	Function	Product Type
DGAC Scientific Report	500+-page *2015 DGAC Scientific Report*	Secretaries of USDA and HHS	To synthesize the evidence base for developing the *DGA* recommendations	Science-based technical report, including background, rationale, and analysis
DGA Policy Report	100-page *2015–2020 DGA*	Federal staff, health professionals, policy makers, industry	To convey scientific and policy-related information supporting the *DGA* recommendations to fulfill the National Nutrition Monitoring and Related Research Act	A report centered on the *DGA* recommendations per se
***DGA* recommendations**	**"Follow a healthy eating pattern across the life span"**	**General public**	**To provide easy-to-understand nutritional and dietary information for public use**	**Brief, consumer-oriented guidelines that can stand alone or be incorporated into other products of the *DGA* process**
DGA disseminations	"Choose MyPlate"	General public or subsets thereof	To promote implementation of the *DGA* recommendations	Easy-to-understand bulletins, graphics, and others based on the *DGA* recommendations

NOTE: Bold text indicates a proposed addition.

BOX 2-1
Proposed Purpose and Goal Statements for the *Dietary Guidelines for Americans*

Proposed purpose statement for the guidelines:

The purpose of the *DGA* is to provide science-based "nutritional and dietary information and guidelines for the general public" that form the basis for "any federal food, nutrition, or health program" (based on the National Nutrition Monitoring and Related Research Act).

Goals of the guidelines:

1. Promote dietary intake that helps improve health and reduce the risk of chronic disease.
2. Provide the federal government with a consistent approach for nutrition policy and messaging.

To achieve the promise of the *DGA*, this National Academies committee proposes that the *DGA* adhere to a consistent set of purposes and goals across cycles, based on the National Nutrition Monitoring and Related Research Act (such as those seen in Box 2-1).

FINDINGS ABOUT THE PROCESS TO UPDATE THE *DGA*

The process to update the *DGA* has evolved over time to account for advances in nutrition science. However, this National Academies committee found the entire *DGA* process has not been comprehensively reconsidered in a manner that effectively allows it to adapt to change while also protecting the integrity of the process. For example, to keep up to date with improvements in the evidence base, the Nutrition Evidence Library was introduced to conduct original systematic reviews. Although the ability to consider original systematic reviews has led to improvements in the *DGA*, the use of original systematic reviews has also resulted in questions about the validity of the evidence assessments. The following sections summarize the key findings of this National Academies committee as they relate to process cycle time and component tasks, transparency, and participation. A more complete discussion of the process and this National Academies committee's findings and conclusions can be found in Part II of this report.

Opportunities for Improving Cycle Time and Component Tasks

The *DGA* have traditionally followed a paradigm where the entire *DGA* are reviewed with each 5-year cycle. However, similar findings and messages have been repeated over the history of the *DGA*. Moreover, several of the *DGA* recommendations have been quite stable over a number of cycles (see Appendix D), bringing into question the utility and effectiveness of reviewing large portions of the entire body of literature every cycle.

In addition to the 5-year cycle time specified in the National Nutrition Monitoring and Related Research Act, the scientific review conducted by the DGAC is limited to a 2-year term by the Federal Advisory Committee Act.[3] Component tasks related to the DGAC—including identifying topics, requesting analyses be conducted, evaluating the science, and developing conclusions—all need to be completed within the 2-year term limit in order to inform the development of the *DGA Policy Report*. As described in Chapter 5, the 2015 DGAC, which followed a process similar to that of the 2005 and 2010 DGACs, spent one-third of its time (8 out of 24 months) devoted to preliminary work such as understanding the work of the previous DGAC, identifying topics and questions for review, and then waiting for the scientific assessments to be completed. This National Academies committee believes having to finalize all these component tasks in 2 years, while also synthesizing and interpreting the evidence, challenges the quality of the *DGA* updates and constrains opportunities for greater stakeholder participation. The current process would benefit from a redesign that increases time available for stakeholder engagement, evidence assessment, and deliberations, while being responsive to change.

Opportunities for Increased Transparency

Transparency is an important attribute of trustworthy guidelines. The current process to update the *DGA* can be made more transparent. The entire process has not been clearly described, particularly steps related to decision making. For example, how DGAC members and consultants are selected has not been made clear. How federal *DGA* writing team members are selected or what standards it uses when developing the *DGA* recommendations is not thoroughly documented. Additionally, how the writing team interpreted the *DGAC Scientific Report* and why some conclusions were modified or omitted when developing the *DGA Policy Report* has also not been clearly described. This lack of transparency

[3] Per the Federal Advisory Committee Act, discretionary federal advisory committees are limited to 2-year terms, but may be permitted to disband sooner if the work of the committee is complete.

resulted in suggestions that the process is being inappropriately influenced by the food sector, lobbyists, faddism, and the federal government (see Chapter 1). Standards for guideline development now include high levels of transparency and are increasingly being adopted, for example, by the U.S. Preventive Services Task Force and the World Health Organization (Brouwers, 2010; Guyatt et al., 2008; HHS, 2014; IOM, 2011; Schünemann et al., 2013, 2014; WHO, 2017). The current process also does not clearly separate the roles of selecting topics, conducting analyses, interpreting the evidence, and drawing conclusions. This confluence of roles adds to the appearance that decisions may not be made independently throughout the *DGA* process.

Additionally, the secretaries have directed each new cycle of the *DGA* to begin with a DGAC to evaluate the previous version of the *DGAC Scientific Report* and *DGA Policy Report* to determine whether updates of previous conclusions are required. Thereby, each successive DGAC appears to have determined its own direction of inquiry and review in the absence of an explicit, overarching strategic plan that spans multiple cycles of the *DGA*. As a result, the transparency of the process to evaluate and translate the science is suboptimized. The priorities for the scope and shape of future *DGA* have also not been consistent or predictable. The lack of clear documentation and disclosure has led to concerns about the impartiality of the decisions being made.

Opportunities for Increased Participation

Timely, proactive stakeholder engagement is another attribute of effective guidelines. The current process offers several opportunities for stakeholder engagement such as the requests for nominations for DGAC members and comments regarding the *DGAC Scientific Report* (see Chapter 5). USDA and HHS have invited written comments throughout the duration of the DGAC's deliberative process. The public also has had opportunities to make suggestions orally to the DGAC and the federal staff developing the *DGA*. However, more opportunities for public participation exist that may add value and credibility to the process. For example, the public can be provided venues or mechanisms to participate at key steps in the process, such as topic identification and question development.

These findings suggest that a number of opportunities for improvement exist and need to be acted upon to help enhance the integrity of the process to update the *DGA*, suggesting the need for the process to be redesigned.

VALUES TO ENHANCE THE INTEGRITY OF THE PROCESS OF DEVELOPING THE *DGA*

In response to its charge, this National Academies committee envisions an updated, redesigned *DGA* process. The redesigned process would clarify the audiences and purposes of the various reports that result from the *DGA* process, improve efficiencies, and introduce advances in scientific methods used. Together, these changes are expected to improve the integrity of the process for updating the *DGA*.

In its first report, this National Academies committee identified five values for improving the integrity of the process used to select the members of the DGAC:

1. Enhance transparency.
2. Manage biases and conflicts of interest.
3. Promote diversity of expertise and experience.
4. Support a deliberative process.
5. Adopt state-of-the-art processes and methods (NASEM, 2017).

This National Academies committee believes these same values remain applicable to the full process used to update the *DGA*. If operationalized, the values can collectively address the aforementioned opportunities for improvement. The five values have been adapted to apply to the redesign of the *DGA* process and are described in the following sections.

Emanating from these values and the proposed redesign is the concept that a more flexible process can result in more efficient use of resources and a minimization of duplication of efforts, particularly as the needs and topics of the *DGA* evolve (see Box 2-2).

Enhancing Transparency

To produce trustworthy *DGA* and provide assurances that decisions are not tainted by bias or undue influence, the process to produce the *DGA* must be transparent. A fundamental value of the *DGA* process redesign is to enhance transparency of the process. It is a multilayered process that needs to be transparent at each level, requiring each step of the process be documented and updated, and that such documentation be readily available to the public. Documentation of the steps used to evaluate the scientific evidence and to reach consensus on the *DGA* would help the public to more thoroughly understand the complexities of the processes needed to update the *DGA* and potentially lead to greater credibility in the decisions made.

BOX 2-2
Leveraging Existing Resources

USDA and HHS both house agencies that work on issues that overlap with the *DGA*. Many of these resources are already being used to update the *DGA*; for example, research from USDA's Agricultural Research Service and HHS's National Institutes of Health (NIH) and the Centers for Disease Control and Prevention (CDC) were central sources of data used in the development of the *2015–2020 DGA*. However, greater synergies are possible to help advance the science and define the issues. The USDA Food and Nutrition Service administers 15 federal nutrition assistance programs, which all must promote the *DGA*, and it could have a unique perspective in helping define issues for evaluation. The Agricultural Research Service conducts research to assess the nutritional needs of Americans. Within HHS, the Agency for Healthcare Research and Quality conducts systematic reviews through its Evidence-based Practice Center Program. The *DGA* could also use resources from CDC's National Center for Chronic Disease Prevention and Health Promotion to identify data related to chronic diseases. HHS also has numerous activities requiring prioritization of topics, including Healthy People, from which lessons and tools could be learned and adapted.

Other ongoing federal activities exist to help coordinate federal nutrition efforts, such as the Interagency Committee on Human Nutrition Research, with the goal of increasing effectiveness and productivity of federally supported or conducted human nutrition research (NAL, 2017). NIH has established some activities to coordinate nutrition research and discuss research challenges and opportunities, as well as a new initiative to develop a NIH-wide strategic plan for nutrition research (NIDDK, 2017a,b). USDA also hosts the Human Nutrition Coordinating Committee to exchange information and coordinate activities for National Nutrition Month. Specific to the *DGA*, the Dietary Guidance Review Committee helps oversee the review of materials within HHS and USDA to ensure dietary guidance for the public is consistent with the *DGA*, such as information in Choose MyPlate, dietary information disseminated in the Special Supplemental Nutrition Program for Women, Infants, and Children (WIC) program, and toolkits for health professionals. Efforts to disseminate the *DGA* recommendations could build on these federal nutrition education programs, as well as state and local partners, such as extension agents. The roles of these federal groups might need to be restructured as a result of modifications to the *DGA* process.

Managing Biases and Conflicts of Interest to Promote Independence in Decision Making

An effective process redesign needs to ensure independence in decision making. The different steps of the process—topic identification, scientific review, development of *DGA* recommendations—are unique and necessarily involve multiple actors representing different areas of expertise and experience. The process redesign will need to align the roles and responsibilities needed at each step of the process with appropriate experts involved in decision making. As discussed in this National Academies committee's first report, the biases of called-upon experts should be balanced among a broad representation of perspectives. Actual and/or perceived conflicts of interest—both financial and nonfinancial—will need to be eliminated to the extent possible or their effects be minimized and managed (see Box 2-3).

Promoting Diversity of Participation, Expertise, and Experience

Trustworthiness of the process can also be enhanced by increasing participation. This National Academies committee believes a diversity of perspectives (i.e., from a broad range of expertise and experience) needs to be represented and considered at appropriate times throughout the process by which the *DGA* are produced. Opportunities for meaningful public participation and engagement at each step of the process (i.e., topic selection, scientific review, development of *DGA* recommendations) are essential. In the steps of the process where public participation would be inappropriate, such as decision making for the *DGA* recommendations themselves, it will be critical for the agencies responsible for the *DGA* to explain to the public why key decisions were made.

Encouraging participation from stakeholders who represent a wide variety of perspectives, including the public, is also critical to fostering diversity. However, it is important to recognize that not every possible viewpoint has to be or can be represented. In this report, the term stakeholder is used to mean active partners in the process to update the *DGA*, including the general public, academia and researchers, advocacy groups, professional organizations, the food sector,[4] and federal agencies. Different stakeholders have unique roles in advancing the goals of the *DGA*. For example, health professionals and federal agencies can help review the utility of resources developed to disseminate the *DGA* prior to their publication. The food sector can help highlight the implications of specific *DGA* recommendations on the food supply or production.

The transfer of knowledge from science-based recommendations into actionable guidance that may be adopted by the general public can be challenging. An intentional effort to do so is warranted and should be guided by models that deploy proven processes. In the case of the Ottawa Model, the process to transfer research recommendations into practical guidance follows six steps: (1) setting the stage; (2) specifying the innovation; (3) assessing the innovation, potential adopters, and the environment

---

[4] In this report, the term *food sector* is used to refer to food manufacturers, retailers, food service, and restaurants.

BOX 2-3
Considerations for Managing Biases and Conflicts of Interest from *Optimizing the Process to Update the Dietary Guidelines for Americans: The Selection Process*

"Although they are often considered together, bias and conflict of interest are distinct. This National Academies committee considers a bias to be an intellectual predisposition toward a particular perspective and an inherent part of being a subject matter expert. Because bias is intrinsically subjective, it is difficult to identify and measure (Jacobson, 2016). Given this, an advisory committee requiring specific expertise to address its charge cannot be entirely free of biases. Biases are, therefore, something to be managed rather than eliminated."

"Conflicts of interest, in contrast, are 'a set of circumstances that creates a risk that professional judgment or actions regarding a primary interest will be unduly influenced by a secondary interest' (IOM, 2009). Individuals can be influenced by factors that are financial and nonfinancial in nature."

"Assessing conflicts of interest does not mean that an individual's behavior is unethical. Instead, it is intended to identify an unacceptable risk of undue influence. Policies covering conflicts of interest generally do not presume that financial gains or other conflicts necessarily sway an individual's viewpoints (IOM, 2009). Nonfinancial conflicts of interest can be just as, if not more, influential than financial conflicts (Akl et al., 2014; Bero, 2014; Guyatt et al., 2010; IOM, 2009). Additionally, while there is a difference between actual and perceived conflicts, the perception is sometimes enough to promote mistrust."

"But given the breadth of this National Academies committee's definitions of biases and conflicts of interest to include nonfinancial conflicts, the committee does not believe these influences can be eliminated *entirely*. As such, those who have had relationships with industry or issue-specific advocates in the recent past could participate fairly on a panel if the nature of the relationship was incidental to the work of the panel. However, strict policies must be made publicly available explaining how such conflicts will be identified and managed."

"If a conflict exists, depending on the type (financial or nonfinancial) and severity, these three management strategies may be employed:

1. The individual should not serve on the committee (Rowe et al., 2013).
2. The individual should serve on the committee in a limited capacity, but not participate in decision making or voting regarding the recommendation for which they have a conflict (Guyatt et al., 2010; Neumann et al., 2013).
3. The individual should serve on the committee as long as a counter-viewpoint is represented for balance (Viswanathan et al., 2014)."

SOURCE: NASEM, 2017, pp. 9, 52, 83.

for barriers and facilitators; (4) selecting and monitoring the knowledge translation strategies; (5) monitoring innovation adoption; and (6) evaluating outcomes of the innovation (NCCMT, 2010). Although a more in-depth discussion of knowledge transfer is beyond the scope of this report, this National Academies committee believes there is significant value in considering a formal approach to translate and transfer knowledge into practical guidance for the public.

Encouraging adoption of the *DGA* could be facilitated by including topics of importance to the general public through established methods such as trend analysis of Internet searches and social media (e.g., Google trends, Twitter analytics, news media sources) and surveys. Once true trends are identified, analytical techniques such as data mining and geospatial information mapping can be used to determine what topics are of interest to the general public, as well as to subpopulations. Surveys could also be conducted to identify what nutrition topics are of public interest. To develop guidelines that people can follow, it will be important to turn the *DGA* recommendations into practical advice to help consumers make decisions in the marketplace.

While broad participation in the process should be proactively sought, participation needs to be incorporated thoughtfully. For example, in addition to specific calls for comments regarding DGAC membership, participation also ought to be incorporated in other steps of the process, such as topic identification. The use of technical experts throughout the process is another way to engage with interested parties. Invited experts could be members of or called upon by a federal advisory committee to share ideas or respond to concepts, or serve as peer reviewers. As discussed in this National Academies committee's first report, care will need to be taken to account for potential biases and conflicts of interest. All stakeholders could provide input into the process; however, only experts as appointed by the secretaries of USDA and HHS ought to be involved in decision-making processes throughout the development of the *DGA*, including the *DGA Policy Report*.

Supporting a More Deliberative Process

Another value of the process redesign is to support a more deliberative approach that is adaptive to dynamic shifts in the system in which it operates. Characteristics of a deliberative process include supporting adaptability, continuity, and continuous learning. The redesign seeks to adopt a more deliberative process by obtaining input from multiple stakeholders, as discussed above, and by adopting a process that is adaptable to changing circumstances. Although the present process for establishing the *DGA* results in a report once in every 5-year cycle, the committee believes that a more continuous model, with deliberations by different constituent committees during the cycle, would be advantageous. This redesign would increase continuity from cycle to cycle and would incorporate continuous quality improvement into the process. Deliberations would go on at various stages of the process, assuring greater input from experts, generalists, stakeholders, and the public at large.

Increasing Adaptability and Flexibility

One characteristic of a deliberative process to update the *DGA* is responsiveness to the needs of stakeholders, including the nutrition community, technical experts, and the public. To that end, the process needs to be flexible enough to recognize the rapidly changing environment of diet and health, and the process needs to progressively move closer to elucidating the complex systems involved. As a result, the *DGA* process could shift from operating as a deterministic structure to one that has the agility to adapt to change and address high-priority topics in detail.

After review and discussion, this National Academies committee believes that the secretaries of USDA and HHS have flexibility in interpreting the National Nutrition Monitoring and Related Research Act and are able to adopt a more flexible process for reviewing, updating, and publishing the *DGA*. Given how the purpose and audience of the *DGA* have changed over time, the breadth and content of each required report ought to be interpreted such that *not all topics* require a detailed review every 5 years. Brief updates of evidence may be conducted, or a particular *DGA* recommendation could be extended and continued without a new in-depth review, unless ongoing surveillance (as described in Chapters 4 and 6) suggests that specific topics need to be restudied. Continually updating the *DGA* recommendations will necessarily be a time-intensive, difficult process to conduct, but precedent has been set for guidelines having an "expiration date" or sunset clause (APA, 2015; Graham and Harrison, 2005; IOM, 2011). For *DGA* recommendations for which the strength of evidence is very strong, the expiration date could be longer than those for which the evidence is rated as moderate. Resulting changes would be made with consideration of the full set of *DGA* recommendations.

In a redesigned process where only portions of the *DGA* are updated in each cycle, only those topics with enough data to generate a full review would be considered for inclusion in the next *DGA* cycle, which would also allow for a broader range of topics to be considered. Topics for review could include those that (1) have been reviewed previously and a body of new evidence now exists; (2) have met their expiration date; or (3) are new and being considered for inclusion in the *DGA* for the first time. The resulting process would likely be more resource efficient than the current process. Additionally, for end users, a more flexible process might produce a *DGA* that is easier to implement, by virtue of limiting the recommendations to changes from the previous edition.

Improving Continuity

To facilitate a deliberative process, the *DGA* cycles need to be considered as a continuous activity to foster learning across cycles. In this way, the body of evidence describing the relationship between diet and health can progressively grow, instead of providing static recommendations that are relevant only for a given 5-year cycle or leaving the impression with the general public that recommendations change frequently. By building on identified gaps in knowledge between *DGA* cycles to develop and prioritize questions for consideration, the effectiveness, efficiency, and transparency of the process can be improved.

Explicitly integrating a process linkage between *DGA* cycles entails making large structural changes, and must be approached deliberately to minimize unintended consequences. To guide a restructuring effort, this National Academies committee believes continuity needs to be integral to the *DGA* process to develop a more strategic approach to accomplish the goals and vision of the *DGA*. Development of such an approach can help provide additional opportunities for stakeholder participation and increase transparency of what is included in the *DGAC Scientific Report* and the *DGA Policy Report*, and can shape the scope of future *DGA* in more predictable ways.

Assuring Continuous Learning

The *DGA* process itself needs to evolve and improve dynamically in order to achieve its goals. This is a consequence of the speed of change in science and evidence generation, as well as continuous introduction of new information and communication technologies. A continuous quality improvement system needs to be developed and implemented to meet this requirement, and was recommended previously in Chapter 5 of this National Academies committee's first report in the context of improving the subprocess for selecting the DGAC committee: "Recommendation 4. The secretaries of USDA and HHS should adopt a system for continuous process improvement to enhance outcomes and performance of the Dietary Guidelines Advisory Committee selection process" (NASEM, 2017, p. 92). That recommendation also applies to the process to update the *DGA*.

Continuous quality improvement requires a long-term commitment and the resources to appropriately collect and evaluate data, report back to relevant stakeholders, and engage with them in iterative cycles of improvement. Data for evaluating the overall process could be collected to measure the level and nature of stakeholder participation, as well as levels of satisfaction among experts involved with developing the *DGA* after implementation of the process redesign. Transparent and participatory continuous quality improvement can also help improve the integrity of the *DGA* process.

To best assess the growth and the adequacy of the process to update the *DGA*, the secretaries of USDA and HHS will need to implement a monitoring and evaluation plan as soon as possible. The term *monitor* as used here generally refers to a set of activities to systematically track progress of the implementation of a process. Ongoing monitoring of the short- and long-term adoption and effect of the *DGA* can help inform future updates. For example, knowing the rates of adherence to the *DGA*, the reasons for nonadherence, and related trends by populations could be helpful in being able to target how messages are crafted and disseminated in future cycles. Data from market trends databases and consumer behavior and values surveys could also be considered. Progress in filling research gaps through federal research initiatives such as the validation of chronic disease biomarkers, among others, also could be monitored to help advance the state of the evidence.

Evaluations build on monitoring activities and focus on analyzing the overall process and its effect. Understanding the effect of the *DGA* on federal food assistance and nutrition education and outreach programs will be important for assessing the overall effectiveness and relevance of the *DGA*. For example, have changes in adherence been observed in those enrolled in the WIC program and children in the school foods program? Other ways to measure adherence to the *DGA* include reviewing food intakes. The National Health and Nutrition Examination Survey estimates usual dietary distribution intakes of *individual* nutrients, foods, and food groups included in the *DGA*; these analyses are routinely conducted and have been provided to the DGAC in the past as described in Chapter 6. One way to assess adherence to the *entire set* of *DGA* recommendations is through the Healthy Eating Index, which is designed to measure conformance to the *DGA* through survey data and has been updated after each of the past three *DGA* cycles. Healthy Eating Index scores and component scores can be used to identify different patterns of eating. These scores could be applied not only at the level of individual diets but also to foods consumed in the marketplace or restaurants, or even the national food supply.

In the long term, the effectiveness and efficiency of the process will need to be assessed. For example, it was hypothesized that introducing strategic planning and flexibility into the process would simplify each successive *DGA* cycle. Determining whether the costs and time associated with implementing the process are appropriate will also be a valuable indicator of the success of the process.

Adopting State-of-the-Art Processes and Methods to Maximize Scientific Rigor

Scientific disciplines evolve and adapt with the emergence of new evidence. To maximize scientific rigor, the process by which the science is reviewed needs to be strengthened by using (1) validated, standardized processes and methods, as available; and (2) the most up-to-date data from nutrition monitoring surveys, food databases, and disease surveillance systems. Processes and actions ought to be based on the best available evidence, requiring that the quality of the current types of evidence (i.e., systematic reviews, food pattern modeling, and data analysis) be continuously improved. In situations where data are owned by the food sector, the companies could be sourced for inclusion. Chapter 4 offers specific suggestions for strengthening these analyses.

An emerging scientific discipline and suite of methods that can be applied in nutrition is systems science (Lee et al., 2017). Systems approaches and methods aim at elucidating the interactions and pathways (e.g., biological, behavioral, social, and environmental) involved in complex relationships, such as the relationship between diet and health. Systems methods can elucidate the dynamic behavior of a system and can help generate hypotheses to explain why a system acts in certain ways. Systems science has been successfully used in other fields such as weather and transportation, and there have been calls to use systems science to address nutrition-related problems such as obesity (Maglio et al., 2014). Although the integration of systems approaches in the field of nutrition is still in its infancy, these approaches hold a lot of promise. With respect to the *DGA*, establishing and modeling the multisectoral relationships and pathways between diet and health has the potential to strengthen the science base of the *DGA* recommendations and can identify important gaps that require further investigation. Systems methods can also help identify and explain the probable limitations of the *DGA* and illustrate what effect can be expected from dietary changes in alternative scenarios.

The *DGA* can play a key role in advancing the understanding of the role of diet within the larger system of factors that affect health. However, understanding the precise role of each *DGA* recommendation in improving health and reducing chronic disease risk is a long-term iterative process that will take multiple *DGA* cycles to complete, but over time will lead to increasing clarity. When systems approaches are fully integrated into the *DGA* process, systems maps and models can continue to evolve to reflect new evidence and move toward better representing the mechanisms and pathways involved. Integrating systems approaches into the evidence review process will be useful to advance the understanding of the potential contribution and limits of the *DGA* to improving health and reducing the risk of chronic disease. Additionally, supporting and conducting studies to evaluate and test the nature of the *DGA*'s contribution is an important component of an effective continually improving process. It is the belief of this National Academies committee that systems approaches could develop into an essential tool for understanding the many dynamic interactions and mechanisms by which diet affects health. These tools could be applied with a goal of improving health. Further discussion regarding the actual methods of systems science can be found in Chapter 4.

BROADENING THE SCOPE OF THE *DGA*

A fundamental change is required such that future cycles of the *DGA* focus on the general public across the entire life span, and not just healthy Americans ages 2 years and older. The Agricultural Act of 2014 mandates that the *2020–2025 DGA* include considerations for pregnant women and children from birth to 24 months (see Chapter 5 for more details). Given the prevalence of chronic disease and risk for chronic disease in the population, this National Academies committee believes it will also be essential for the *DGA Policy Report* to include all Americans whose health can benefit by improving their diet based on the scientific evidence. Without these changes, present and future dietary guidance will not be applicable to a large majority of the general population.

Numerous organizations including the National Institutes of Health and professional societies have developed and endorsed their own population- or disease-specific dietary guidelines. The *DGA* are not designed to adjudicate among the various dietary guidelines, but confusion regarding these multiple sets of guidelines could be reduced. One way to help the public understand which set of dietary guidelines to follow would be to identify areas of consistency among the various guidelines that are developed in a manner consistent with the methods used in the *DGA*; these other guidelines could be referred to in the *DGA Policy Report*.

Specific to those who have an established disease, making good dietary choices is part of managing disease and controlling chronic disease risk factors. In some cases, disease prevention or treatment is primarily dietary, while in others diet is part of a more complex plan of management. Whereas a movement toward encompassing persons with chronic disease as the intended audience for the *DGA* is at present aspirational, one example with strong evidence is the Dietary Approaches to Stop Hypertension (DASH) dietary pattern. The DASH dietary pattern is prominently recommended as part of a healthful eating pattern for those with hypertension and prehypertension (NIH, 2015) and is consistent with the *DGA* recommendations. Such high standards of evidence are needed to be able to address disease management. As the evidence base increases, opportunities need to be capitalized on to provide dietary recommendations that address management of other diseases.

If the focus of the *DGA* is shifted to include the general public, such a shift will likely have many implications for the process of establishing the *DGA*, the *DGA* themselves, as well as associated eating patterns. For example, an eating pattern for weight loss might need to emphasize where calories could be reduced without compromising the nutritional quality of the diet. A diet for secondary prevention of heart disease might be based on an eating pattern recommended for the general public, but include specific modifications known to decrease the risk of cardiac events in those individuals with heart disease. Providing more information on eating patterns could help enable health care providers in their use of the *DGA*. Additionally, broadening the scope of the *DGA* will bring challenges and likely require new approaches to evaluate the evidence. For instance, research on the effect of diet exposures in pregnancy and early life on long-term disease risk is a relatively new field predominated by observational studies. New approaches to evaluation of such data need to be developed. The *DGA* always needs to be based on the best available evidence using a variety of methods (see Chapter 4 for further discussion). The process redesign will provide opportunities to expand the methodological approaches to develop the *DGA* to include broader groups of people with a range of physiological needs, metabolic health, and chronic disease states.

CONCLUSION

The *DGA* can play a role in improving health and reducing the risk of chronic disease in America, and can greatly affect the foods and combinations of foods that people consume. However, the effect of the *DGA* will be limited if they do not apply to the general population and if the public questions the credibility of the process and the ultimate *DGA* recommendations. To develop a trustworthy *DGA*, the process needs to be redesigned. USDA and HHS have the opportunity to adopt a more flexible, continuous process that engages a broad stakeholder community in the *DGA* process. It will be imperative for the process to enhance transparency, manage biases and conflicts of interest to promote independent decision making, promote diversity of expertise and experience, support a deliberative process, and adopt state-of-the-art processes and methods to maximize scientific rigor. A process redesign model is proposed in Chapter 3.

REFERENCES

Akl, E. A., P. El-Hachem, H. Abou-Haidar, I. Neumann, H. J. Schünemann, and G. H. Guyatt. 2014. Considering intellectual, in addition to financial, conflicts of interest proved important in a clinical practice guideline: A descriptive study. *Journal of Clinical Epidemiology* 67(11):1222-1228.

APA (American Psychological Association). 2015. Professional practice guidelines: Guidance for developers and users. *American Psychologist* 70(9):823-831.

Bero, L. 2014. What is in a name? Nonfinancial influences on the outcomes of systematic reviews and guidelines. *Journal of Clinical Epidemiology* 67(11):1239-1241.

Brouwers, M., M. E. Kho, G. P. Browman, J. S. Burgers, F. Cluzeau, G. Feder, B. Fervers, I. D. Graham, J. Grimshaw, S. Hanna, P. Littlejohns, J. Makarski, and L. Zitzelsberger, for the AGREE Next Steps Consortium. 2010. AGREE II: Advancing guideline development, reporting and evaluation in healthcare. *Canadian Medical Association Journal* 182(18):E839-E842.

CDC (Centers for Disease Control and Prevention). 1998. Recommendations to prevent and control iron deficiency in the United States. *Morbidity and Mortality Weekly Report. Recommendations and Reports* 47(Rr-3):1-29.

Erdrich, J., X. Zhang, E. Giovannucci, and W. Willett. 2015. Proportion of colon cancer attributable to life style in a cohort of U.S. women. *Cancer Causes & Control* 26(9):1271-1279.

Graham, I. D., and M. B. Harrison. 2005. Evaluation and adaptation of clinical practice guidelines. *Evidence-Based Nursing* 8(3):68-72.

Guyatt, G. H., A. D. Oxman, R. Kunz, Y. Falck-Ytter, G. E. Vist, A. Liberati, and H. J. Schünemann. 2008. Going from evidence to recommendations. *BMJ* 336(7652):1049-1051.

Guyatt, G., E. A. Akl, J. Hirsh, C. Kearon, M. Crowther, D. Gutterman, S. Z. Lewis, I. Nathanson, R. Jaeschke, and H. Schünemann. 2010. The vexing problem of guidelines and conflict of interest: A potential solution. *Annals of Internal Medicine* 152(11):738-741.

HHS (U.S. Department of Health and Human Services). 2014. Open government plan: Version 3.0. https://wayback.archive-it.org/org-745/20170703163931/https://www.hhs.gov/sites/default/files/open/plan/open-gov-plan-v3.pdf (accessed August 16, 2017).

HHS/USDA (U.S. Department of Agriculture). 2015. Dietary Guidelines for Americans *2015 – 2020: Eighth edition*. https://health.gov/dietaryguidelines/2015/guidelines (accessed July 18, 2017).

Hill, J. O., H. R. Wyatt, and J. C. Peters. 2012. Energy balance and obesity. *Circulation* 126(1):126-132.

IOM (Institute of Medicine). 2001. *Dietary Reference Intakes for vitamin A, vitamin K, arsenic, boron, chromium, copper, iodine, iron, manganese, molybdenum, nickel, silicon, vanadium, and zinc.* Washington, DC: National Academy Press.

IOM. 2009. *Conflict of interest in medical research, education, and practice.* Washington, DC: The National Academies Press.

IOM. 2011. *Clinical practice guidelines we can trust.* Washington, DC: The National Academies Press.

Jacobson, P. 2016 (unpublished). Approaches to bias and conflict of interest—how would you suggest minimizing conflicts of interest and "eliminating bias" while preserving a wide range of viewpoints. Presentation to the Committee to Review the Process to Update the Dietary Guidelines for Americans, Washington, DC, October 17, 2016.

Krebs-Smith, S. M., P. M. Guenther, A. F. Subar, S. I. Kirkpatrick, and K. W. Dodd. 2010. Americans do not meet federal dietary recommendations. *Journal of Nutrition* 140(10):1832-1838.

Lee, B. Y., S. M. Bartsch, Y. Mui, L. A. Haidari, M. L. Spiker, and J. Gittelsohn. 2017. A systems approach to obesity. *Nutrition Reviews* 75(Suppl 1):94-106.

Maglio, P. P., M. J. Sepulveda, and P. L. Mabry. 2014. Mainstreaming modeling and simulation to accelerate public health innovation. *American Journal of Public Health* 104(7):1181-1186.

NAL (National Agriculture Library). 2017. *Interagency Committee on Human Nutrition Research*. Beltsville, MD: U.S. Department of Agriculture. https://www.nal.usda.gov/fnic/interagency-committee-human-nutrition-research (accessed May 31, 2017).

NASEM (National Academies of Sciences, Engineering, and Medicine). 2017. *Optimizing the process for establishing the* Dietary Guidelines for Americans: *The selection process*. Washington, DC: The National Academies Press.

NCCMT (National Collaborating Centre for Methods and Tools). 2010. *Ottawa model of research use: A framework for adopting innovations*. Hamilton, ON: McMaster University.

Neumann, I., R. Karl, A. Rajpal, E. A. Akl, and G. H. Guyatt. 2013. Experiences with a novel policy for managing conflicts of interest of guideline developers: A descriptive qualitative study. *Chest* 144(2):398-404.

Nicklas, T. A., L. Jahns, M. L. Bogle, D. N. Chester, M. Giovanni, D. M. Klurfeld, K. Laugero, Y. Liu, S. Lopez, and K. L. Tucker. 2013. Barriers and facilitators for consumer adherence to the *Dietary Guidelines for Americans*: The HEALTH study. *Journal of the Academy of Nutrition and Dietetics* 113(10):1317-1331.

NIDDK (National Institute of Diabetes and Digestive and Kidney Diseases). 2017a. *Nutrition Research Coordinating Committee*. https://www.niddk.nih.gov/about-niddk/advisory-coordinating-committees/nutrition-research-coordinating-committee/Pages/default.aspx (accessed May 31, 2017).

NIDDK. 2017b. *Nutrition Research Task Force*. https://www.niddk.nih.gov/about-niddk/advisory-coordinating-committees/nih-nutrition-research-task-force/Pages/default.aspx (accessed May 31, 2017).

NIH (National Institutes of Health). 2015. *Health benefits of the DASH eating plan*. https://www.nhlbi.nih.gov/health/health-topics/topics/dash/benefits (accessed July 14, 2017).

NRC (National Research Council). 1989. *Diet and health: Implications for reducing chronic disease risk*. Washington, DC: National Academy Press.

Rowe, S., N. Alexander, C. M. Weaver, J. T. Dwyer, C. Drew, R. S. Applebaum, S. Atkinson, F. M. Clydesdale, E. Hentges, N. A. Higley, and M. E. Westring. 2013. How experts are chosen to inform public policy: Can the process be improved? Health Policy 112(3):172-178.

Schünemann, H., J. Brožek, G. Guyatt, and A. Oxman, editors. 2013. *Handbook for grading the quality of evidence and the strength of recommendations using the GRADE approach*. The GRADE Working Group. http://gdt.guidelinedevelopment.org/app/handbook/handbook.html#h.33qgws879zw (accessed August 3, 2017).

Schünemann, H., W. Wiercioch, I. Etxeandia, M. Falavigna, N. Santesso, R. Mustafa, M. Ventresca, R. Brignardello-Petersen, K.-T. Laisaar, S. Kowalski, T. Baldeh, Y. Zhang, U. Raid, I. Neumann, S. L. Norris, J. Thornton, R. Harbour, S. Treweek, G. Guyatt, P. Alonso-Coello, M. Reinap, J. Brožek, A. Oxman, and E. A. Akl. 2014. Guidelines 2.0: Systematic development of a comprehensive checklist for a successful guideline enterprise. *Canadian Medical Association Journal* 186(3):E123-E142.

Stampfer, M. J., F. B. Hu, J. E. Manson, E. B. Rimm, and W. C. Willett. 2000. Primary prevention of coronary heart disease in women through diet and lifestyle. *New England Journal of Medicine* 343(1):16-22.

U.S. Congress, House of Representatives, Committee on Agriculture. 2015. *Hearing to review the development of the 2015* Dietary Guidelines for Americans. 114th Cong., 1st Sess. October 7, 2015.

Viswanathan, M., T. S. Carey, S. E. Belinson, E. Berliner, S. M. Chang, E. Graham, J.-M. Guise, S. Ip, M. A. Maglione, D. C. McCrory, M. McPheeters, S. J. Newberry, P. Sista, and C. M. White. 2014. A proposed approach may help systematic reviews retain needed expertise while minimizing bias from nonfinancial conflicts of interest. *Journal of Clinical Epidemiology* 67(11):1229-1238.

Welsh, S., C. Davis, and A. Shaw. 1992. A brief history of food guides in the United States. *Nutrition Today* 27(6):6-11.

WHO (World Health Organization). 2003. *Diet, nutrition and the prevention of chronic diseases: Report of a joint WHO/FAO expert consultation.* Geneva, Switzerland: World Health Organization (WHO technical report series 916).

WHO. 2017. *Normative work in nutrition at WHO: Priority setting for guideline development.* Geneva, Switzerland: World Health Organization.

Wilson, M. M., J. Reedy, and S. M. Krebs-Smith. 2016. American diet quality: Where it is, where it is heading, and what it could be. *Journal of the Academy of Nutrition and Dietetics* 116(2):302-310.

3

Process Redesign

This National Academies of Sciences, Engineering, and Medicine (the National Academies) committee considers that process redesign for updating the *Dietary Guidelines for Americans* (*DGA*)[1] can improve transparency and stakeholder engagement, accelerate access to expertise and experience, promote independence in decision making, and enhance scientific rigor. If successfully implemented, these changes collectively have the potential to improve trustworthiness of the process to update the *DGA*. Redesign can also improve the agility of the process and provide for continuity of focus in key operational and strategic areas over multiple *DGA* cycles. For example, the *DGA* objective to promote health requires the engagement of many resources and an expanded set of multidisciplinary experts. Redesign that allows for on-demand acquisition of such resources can improve the efficiency of the process (e.g., specialized expertise in behavioral and implementation science, data science, technology, complex systems methods). Redesign can also address needs for improved continuity between *DGA* cycles in operational areas such as real-time monitoring and curation of new evidence, and maintaining a focus on strategic objectives that may span multiple *DGA* cycles.

A more agile and effective process can improve the relevance and usefulness of the *DGA* recommendations. The *DGA* cycle time has been 5 years per the National Nutrition Monitoring and Related Research

---

[1] Refer to Chapter 1, Box 1-1, for an explanation of how the term *DGA* is used throughout this National Academies report.

Act. However, the process to update the *DGA* has occurred over a 3-year time period: 2 years for the work of the Dietary Guidelines Advisory Committee (DGAC), and 1 year for the generation of the *DGA Policy Report*. The remaining 2 years have been voids before the 3-year process is repeated. This National Academies committee believes that using the entire 5 years would provide the opportunity for redesigning the *DGA* process to become more agile, flexible, and effective. The model discussed below accomplishes these objectives by reducing the administrative and operational tasks of the DGAC. This is achieved by redistributing DGAC tasks to provide more time and dedicated expertise to focus on each task in the process.

Recommendation 1. The secretaries of the U.S. Department of Agriculture (USDA) and the U.S. Department of Health and Human Services (HHS) should redesign the *Dietary Guidelines for Americans* (*DGA*) process to prioritize topics to be reviewed in each *DGA* cycle, and redistribute the current functions of the Dietary Guidelines Advisory Committee to three separate groups:

a. Dietary Guidelines Planning and Continuity Group to monitor and curate evidence generation, to identify and prioritize topics for inclusion in the *DGA*, and to provide strategic planning support across *DGA* cycles;

b. Technical expert panels to provide content and methodological consultation during evaluation of the evidence; and

c. Dietary Guidelines Scientific Advisory Committee to interpret the scientific evidence and draw conclusions.

MODEL PROCESS REDESIGN

The following process redesign model retains the components and subprocesses used for the *2015–2020 DGA*, and reflects elements of the process instituted for the review of evidence targeted to pregnancy and infancy that began in 2012 (USDA, 2017). However, the proposed redesign redistributes the tasks among a revised set of groups instead of having all tasks supporting the scientific assessment being conducted by a single group (DGAC). Compared to the current process, separating the tasks allows for more targeted, dedicated expertise to complete a specific task, higher-quality inputs into the synthesis of evidence, and more time for deliberations, stakeholder engagement, and transparency-related activities. This redesign also permits much of the context setting and evidence development to be accomplished early in the process.

In the process redesign model, a Dietary Guidelines Planning and Continuity Group (DGPCG) is established to monitor new relevant scientific evidence, to identify topics and questions for review by the Dietary Guidelines Scientific Advisory Committee (DGSAC), as well as to provide support for DGSAC alignment with any strategic objectives that may span multiple cycles. Subcommittees would be convened as needed to address specific topic areas. The new DGPCG is envisioned to operate continually across *DGA* cycles, but would act primarily in the period before a DGSAC is convened and after the *DGA Policy Report* is updated. The redesign also creates an additional framework to improve support for the scientific needs of the process: technical expert panels (TEPs). The synthesis and interpretation of evidence and the development of conclusions would be the primary focus of the DGSAC. Each of these three entities is discussed in detail below. It will be important for some level of coordination to occur among the group. However, this National Academies committee believes that in order for the proposed redesign to be successfully implemented, specific details (e.g., how each entity operates and coordinates with each other) needs to be left to the secretaries of USDA and HHS and/or the entities themselves to decide.

The model process redesign is shown in Figure 3-1. It displays the new redesigned process as well as the current process on the 5-year *DGA* update timeline. This process redesign model will be referred to throughout the description of the proposed structure and workflow.

The following sections present the roles of each group. Composition of each group is also proposed and is summarized in Table 3-1.

Roles and Composition of the Dietary Guidelines Planning and Continuity Group (DGPCG)

The DGPCG is envisioned as a group of nonfederal experts and several federal staff convened to do the following:

1. Provide the secretaries of USDA and HHS with planning support that assures alignment with long-term strategic objectives spanning multiple *DGA* cycles;
2. Identify and prioritize topics for the DGSAC to evaluate in subsequent *DGA* cycles; and
3. Oversee monitoring and surveillance for new evidence.

Strategic planning is needed across *DGA* cycles to introduce new, relevant topics while also ensuring that all *DGA* recommendations remain based on appropriate scientific evidence. As discussed in Chapter 2, not all topics need to be fully reevaluated every 5 years. The DGPCG would

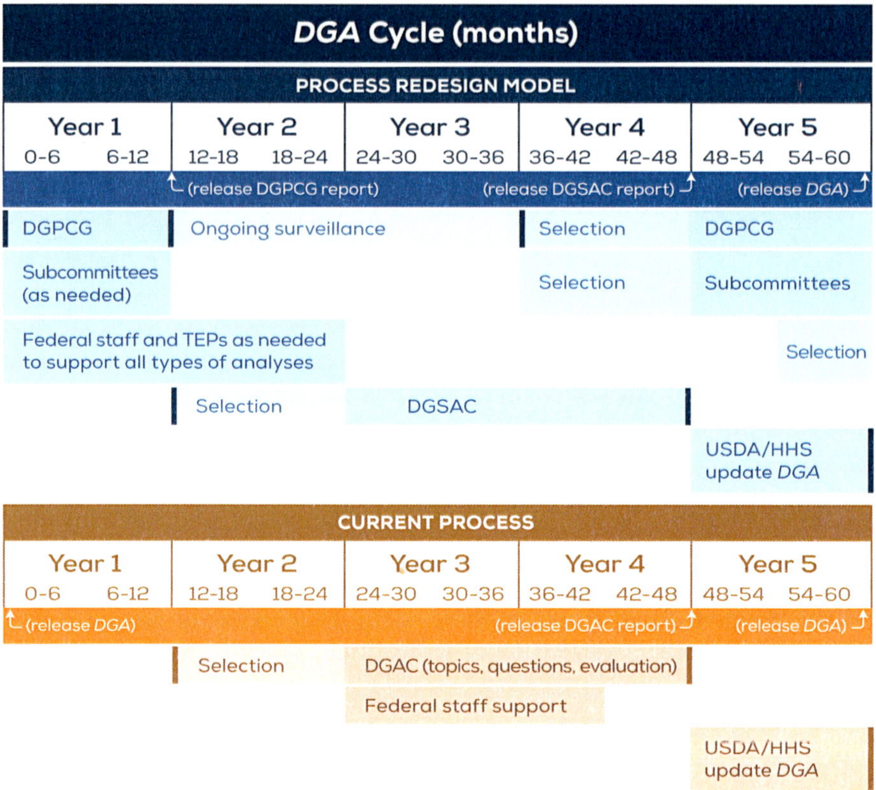

FIGURE 3-1 Proposed timeline for future *DGA* cycles.
NOTES: Dark bars indicate opportunities for public comment and explanation of key decisions made. Darker shaded boxes indicate most active periods, while lighter shaded boxes denote potential times of less active engagement as needed. "Selection" refers to the selection of members for the respective groups. "Federal staff" includes those providing technical support such as the Nutrition Evidence Library staff and those conducting food pattern modeling and descriptive data analyses. *DGA* = *Dietary Guidelines for Americans*; DGAC = Dietary Guidelines Advisory Committee; DGPCG = Dietary Guidelines Planning and Continuity Group; DGSAC = Dietary Guidelines Scientific Advisory Committee; HHS = U.S. Department of Health and Human Services; TEP = technical expert panel; USDA = U.S. Department of Agriculture.

be responsible for publicly disclosing in a brief report the criteria and logic for how it prioritized topics and the associated research questions recommended. The DGPCG would also help to make the process agile. For example, by helping oversee activities to monitor the scientific and public health literature, the DGPCG can assist with determining when

TABLE 3-1 Composition of Groups in the Proposed Process to Update the *DGA*

Group	Function	General Types of Expertise	Specific Types of Proficiencies
Dietary Guidelines Planning and Continuity Group (DGPCG)	• Support strategic planning • Identify, select, and prioritize topics • Oversee monitoring of new evidence	• Half generalists • Half specialists • Nonfederal experts and federal staff	• Broad and specialized nutrition expertise • Federal agency operations • Methodologists (e.g., systematic reviews, systems modeling)
Subcommittees as needed	• Address specific topic areas	• Subject-matter expertise	• Individuals with specific nutrition and/or medical expertise
Technical expert panels (TEPs)			
Systematic reviews	• Help NEL refine key questions, prioritize questions, and establish PICO criteria about a specific topic (e.g., P/B–24, CVD)	• Domain expertise • Methodologic expertise	• Experts in nutrition, health outcomes, public health, general research methods, *and* stakeholders of specific topic being addressed
Other types of analyses	• Help USDA/HHS data team identify and analyze data, prior to convening of DGSAC	• Methodologic expertise	• Data scientists familiar with the relevant methods and data sources
Dietary Guidelines Scientific Advisory Committee (DGSAC)	• Assess systematic reviews and other types of evidence to develop conclusions for USDA/HHS consideration • Identify new questions and topics if needed and seek TEP to assist • Identify topics for DGPCG to consider for the next DGSAC	• Domain expertise • Methodologic expertise	• Experts in methods used and guideline development

NOTE: CVD = cardiovascular disease; HHS = U.S. Department of Health and Human Services; NEL = Nutrition Evidence Library; P/B–24 = pregnant women and children from birth to 24 months; PICO = population, intervention/exposure, comparator, outcome of interest; USDA = U.S. Department of Agriculture.

enough new evidence has been developed on a specific topic to warrant review for potential inclusion in a future *DGA* cycle. The threshold for what constitutes "enough new evidence" ought to be an initial task of the DGPCG and updated as needed. The functions of supporting strategic planning and overseeing monitoring and surveillance for new evidence require that the DGPCG not be time limited and that it operate across *DGA* cycles.

The DGPCG will need to be composed of nongovernmental experts together with federal staff from USDA and HHS to fulfill its mission. Nongovernmental experts would include generalists in nutrition, experts in relevant stages of the life cycle, and experts in core competency areas such as research methods, public health, medicine, implementation science, and food production. The federal staff provide the governmental context and knowledge of the requirements of the federal food and nutrition programs. These core competencies can be supplemented by additional expertise required at any point through various mechanisms, ranging from membership on the DGPCG to advisors. It is envisioned that DGPCG members would serve across 5-year *DGA* cycles, rotating through staggered terms that could begin or end in the middle of a *DGA* cycle. It is the intent of this National Academies committee to leave the secretaries of USDA and HHS the flexibility to determine the size, expertise, member tenure, and ad hoc mechanisms for supplementing DGPCG intelligence needs, as well as the roles of the members themselves. However, the composition of the DGPCG should be selected based on the values and processes delineated in this National Academies committee's first report, including identification and management of potential financial and nonfinancial conflicts of interest (see Boxes 1-4 and 2-3 for further discussion about identifying and managing biases and conflicts of interest).

Supplementing DGPCG Expertise

It is likely that additional expertise will be needed during the deliberations of the DGPCG. For example, fully vetting topic considerations may require expertise not covered by DGPCG members. The DGPCG could seek supplemental expertise in a number of ways, including commissioned papers, invited speakers, consultants or advisors, roundtables, or subcommittees, depending on the breadth and complexity of the topic. Full public access to any form of additional expertise solicited will be needed, and individuals providing such expertise would not be allowed to partake in DGPCG deliberations and decision making. A good model to consider for identifying questions related to topics with broad subject matter is the project to expand the *DGA* to include women who are pregnant and infants and children from birth to 24 months (P/B–24). Specifically, the P/B–24 project engaged with a broad number of stakeholders through both face-to-face workshops and online interactions to identify and develop topics and questions for systematic reviews. The work of the P/B–24 project separated the topic identification process from the evidence evaluation (see Chapter 5 for details).

The extension of the *DGA* to include recommendations for P/B–24 introduced a subpopulation for specific attention and a need for the DGPCG to obtain expertise in these domains on an ongoing basis. The DGPCG will have to consider a broad array of subjects for this demographic group ranging from the developmental needs of infants and varying nutritional requirements of children 0 to 24 months, to feeding behaviors and the roles of caretakers in feeding practices. Because the number of seats on the DGPCG itself will be limited to allow it to be operationally efficient, having experts in each P/B–24 subject is not feasible. A small number of experts in P/B–24 would be members of the DGPCG given the breadth of the subject matter. Additional expertise related to P/B–24 will be required to supplement the DGPCG using any of the aforementioned mechanisms, preferably through appointment of a subcommittee.

Roles and Composition of Technical Expert Panels (TEPs)

TEPs, including nonfederal and federal experts with a diversity of expertise and viewpoints, are proposed by this National Academies committee as a flexible mechanism to supplement the technical insights in beginning stages of any type of evidence analysis. The number and timing of such TEPs will vary based on needs during each *DGA* cycle. It is important to note that TEP members would provide their input on an individual basis; no set of collective advice from the TEP would be prepared. As such, TEPs would not need to convene in person. TEP members would be domain experts well versed in the specific research method being considered. Domain experts are people who are authorities on a specific area or topic. TEP members would be identified by USDA and HHS, and their selection could include consideration of the list of nominees suggested for membership on the DGPCG. Rules for bias and conflicts of interest, as well as scientific positions and views, would need to be created and made publicly available prior to identification.

TEPs would provide content and methodological consultation. For example, a TEP would work with the Nutrition Evidence Library (NEL) in the initial phase of conducting a systematic review. The TEPs would operationalize the research questions formulated by the DGPCG by helping to set the eligibility criteria for the literature review and to clarify systematic review question elements (i.e., population, intervention, comparison, and outcomes). TEPs could also help the NEL with technical issues during the review of the literature by the NEL staff, such as understanding the nuances of measurements, tests, and definitions. A TEP may be convened to provide input on additional systematic review questions identified by a newly constituted DGSAC. TEPs would not be responsible for conducting the systematic review or assessing the quality of the studies. TEP members could also be included in the peer review of the draft systematic review, but if they are, they would only be part of a much larger number of peer reviewers. The use of TEPs is modeled after the inclusion of domain expertise in the Agency for Healthcare Research and Quality (AHRQ) Evidence-based Practice Centers Program and the non-DGAC systematic reviews conducted by the NEL (see Chapter 6 for a full description of how technical experts are used in these processes[2]). In the AHRQ Evidence-based Practice Centers Program, TEPs typically interact with the systematic review team through one to three teleconferences over several weeks to 1 month.

Expert panels could also be employed to supplement the expertise of groups conducting other types of analyses such as food pattern modeling and descriptive data analyses. TEPs for these analyses are envisioned as supporting efforts such as verifying key assumptions in the development of food pattern and systems models or helping refine research questions related to data analyses.

Roles and Composition of the Dietary Guidelines Scientific Advisory Committee (DGSAC)

In the process redesign model, the DGSAC is charged with synthesizing and interpreting scientific evidence, as well as developing conclusions for USDA and HHS to consider in the *DGA* update (see Box 4-2 for descriptions of terminology). Specifically, the DGSAC would be charged with integrating all data inputs such as systematic reviews, food pattern modeling, and descriptive data analyses to develop its conclusions regarding diet and its relationship to health. To evaluate the science, the DGSAC will need to determine a priori the standards of evidence it will consider. As needed, the DGSAC would also be able to identify and request a limited number of new analyses and develop research recommendations for consideration by the DGPCG and the larger research community. The DGSAC would deliver a DGSAC scientific report that would serve as the scientific foundation for the *DGA Policy Report*. The DGSAC would also be charged with identifying topics where more evidence is needed, and

[2] Groups of technical experts are used in the AHRQ Evidence-based Practice Centers Program and the non-DGAC NEL systematic review process. These experts are consulted for their subject-matter expertise and are not considered authors of the final publication.

suggesting those topics for future *DGA* cycles. Owing to the critical nature of this work and the need to ensure integrity of the process, it is essential that the DGSAC provide timely and ample opportunities and forums for stakeholders to provide insights and to engage in transparent and credible ways. However, the DGSAC will act independently in its interpretation of the scientific evidence and in its final conclusions.

As with previous DGACs, members of the DGSAC would include experts in domain subject matters to be reviewed to provide relevant knowledge and context for reviewing the evidence. The DGSAC will also need to include experts in the methods being considered for use in that particular *DGA* cycle (e.g., systematic reviews, food pattern modeling). It will be helpful for DGSAC members to understand best practices for producing guidelines even though the DGSAC will not be crafting the *DGA* recommendations themselves. This knowledge can facilitate creation of effective DGSAC conclusions for the federal *DGA* writing team's consideration in its development of the *DGA Policy Report*. Like the DGPCG, DGSAC members would be selected through the process recommended in this National Academies committee's first report (see Boxes 1-4 and 2-3 for further discussion about identifying and managing biases and conflicts of interest).

Regarding the inclusion of the P/B–24 population, because it is unlikely that this process redesign model could be made fully operational for the *2020–2025 DGA* update, an interim enhancement to the existing process could be developed to add P/B–24-specific expertise to support the DGSAC's synthesis and interpretation of the evidence. To accomplish this, systematic reviews being conducted for the P/B–24 project ought to be peer reviewed, and at least one person with general expertise in the science of P/B–24 and experience with systematic reviews needs to be involved with the DGSAC.

PROPOSED WORKFLOW

At a minimum, this National Academies committee believes the criteria, process, and logic for topic selection and evidence grading must be clearly articulated and fully disclosed. The public, including consumers and stakeholders, need to be provided timely opportunities to engage at key points in the process: (1) nominating topics; (2) responding to a list of selected topics; (3) nominating experts to the DGPCG and DGSAC; (4) commenting on a list of provisional appointees; (5) providing feedback on the DGSAC report; and (6) commenting on the *DGA Policy Report*. While it will not be feasible to engage the public at every task because public comment periods can be lengthy and adds time to the overall process, care should be taken to help build trust in the overall process. The major tasks of the proposed process include topic identification, selection, and prioritization; data collection and evaluation; data synthesis, interpretation, and integration; and the update of the *DGA*.

Topic Identification, Selection, and Prioritization

A critical task in the process to update the *DGA* is deciding on the topics to be reviewed, which can be controversial. To that end, transparency and appropriate opportunities for stakeholder participation are needed to help develop credibility in the final list of topics. A number of procedural decisions will need to be made. For example, will there be an explicit process for making decisions such as putting a voting structure in place? Will methods such as value of information analysis be considered for ranking,[3] or will the process for making decisions be more subjective (i.e., committee discussion and consensus)? Regardless of the process used, it will be necessary to clearly articulate to the public at the onset of the process how topics are identified, selected, and prioritized; the criteria against which topics are considered (see Figure 3-2 for examples); and how the criteria are operationalized. The process for identifying, selecting, and prioritizing topics could be modeled after a number of other processes such as AHRQ's process for comparative effectiveness reviews, Healthy People, and the World Health Organization (Andrews, 2013; HHS, 2008; WHO, 2017).

In the topic identification phase, all stakeholders would nominate topics for potential inclusion in the *DGA*. This National Academies committee believes nominations need to be fielded from a broad group of interested parties, including the public; professional organizations; food sector organizations; researchers; and state, federal, and local governments. Nomination statements ought to have a standard format for purposes of clarity and organization to facilitate selection of potential topics, such as (1) why the topic is important, (2) how the implementation of recommended changes may improve health outcomes, (3) several specific, key questions to explore within the topic, and (4) supporting references as applicable. Topics could be collected by USDA and HHS and then filtered based on explicit criteria, in accordance with a transparent and documented process. In addition, the DGPCG could review topics of public interest even if not specifically nominated, for example through search engine analytics as discussed in Chapter 2. A list of nominated and identi-

[3] Value of information analysis can be used as a tool to set research priorities. It is "an approach to research prioritization which uses Bayesian methods to estimate the potential benefits of gathering further information (through more research) before making a decision" (Myers et al., 2012).

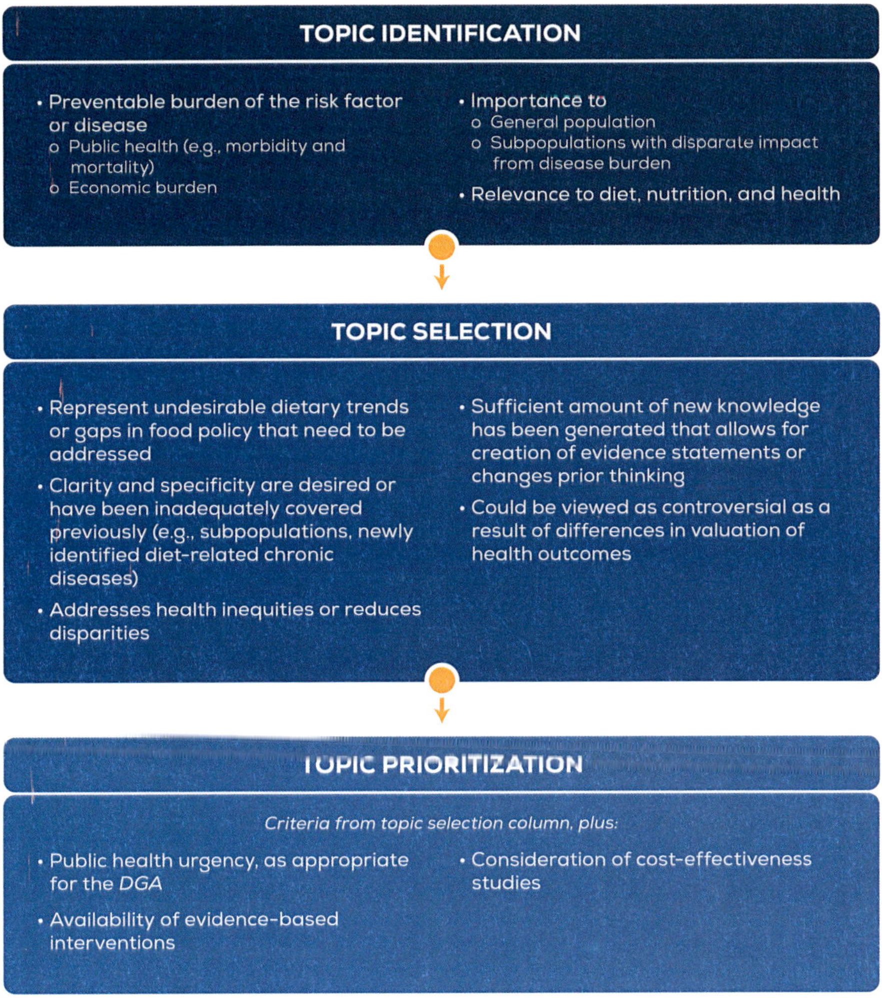

FIGURE 3-2 Examples of criteria for topic identification, selection, and prioritization.
NOTES: These criteria were derived from a number of other efforts at organizations, including the World Health Organization, the Patient-Centered Outcomes Research Institute, the Agency for Healthcare Research and Quality Evidence-based Practice Centers Program, the Institute of Medicine, Cochrane, the U.S. Preventive Services Task Force, the Guide to Community Preventive Services, and the 2015 DGAC. The criteria from each of these organizations were modified to fit the needs of the process to update the *DGA*. The darkest blue box indicates any stakeholder as primary actor; the lighter blue boxes indicate DGPCG as the actor.

fied topics deemed not to be relevant could then be made publicly available. All nominated topics that meet the topic identification criteria ought to be reviewed with the qualification that topics identified as being of strong public interest be of current, not historical, interest. Owing to time and resource constraints, and available evidence, not all topics could be included in each cycle. Topics could be accepted continuously, but cutoff dates could be established for a topic to be considered for each *DGA* cycle.

Topic selection refers to the process for narrowing the list of all relevant nominations to a set of topics eligible to be addressed in the upcoming cycle. In this stage, the DGPCG would consider each identified topic based on a clear set of criteria and would publish a prioritization of selected topics, as well as explanations for why excluded topics or categories of topics were deferred.

The last stage, topic prioritization, refers to the process for choosing the order in which topics are evaluated for inclusion in the *DGA*. The DGPCG could prioritize the topics from the topic selection stage based on its expert opinions and a predetermined set of criteria. The final prioritization would be made publicly available along with a statement of why some topics or a tier of topics were designated as being of lower priority. A lower priority would be designated for the purpose of making evidence gathering feasible, not to indicate that topics be disregarded.

While USDA and HHS proposed criteria for the 2015 DGAC to consider,[4] it is not clear how the DGAC used the criteria. It is this National Academies committee's opinion that specific criteria be clearly defined for each stage and the process by which the criteria are considered be made transparent.

---

[4] The 2015 DGAC was to consider the following draft topic selection criteria: (1) target populations; (2) potential effect on food and nutrition-related outcomes of public health concern, such as health outcomes and diet-related behaviors, and (3) likelihood of informing recommendations, whether it be to suggest new guidance, inform a revision to current guidance, or address urgent public health concerns. Suggested criteria for prioritization included (1) a review of the current evidence on the topic may inform the development of new dietary guidance for Americans ages 2 years and older; (2) a review of the current evidence on the topic may result in a change or elaboration in existing recommendations; (3) the topic represents important uncertainty or a knowledge gap for decision makers; (4) the topic addresses a dilemma in public health nutrition; (5) the topic represents an area where there is a degree of urgency for guidance (e.g., significant area of public health concern, emerging area for public health action); (6) the topic addresses a common practice in public health nutrition for which there is no government guidance; and (7) the topic has the potential to inform the development of dietary guidance that is public health oriented (i.e., the promotion of health and the prevention of disease at the population/community level) and not the development of clinical guidelines to use for the treatment and care of individuals with specific diseases and conditions (see Chapter 5 for details).

Data Collection and Evaluation

As soon as the DGPCG prioritizes topics for a particular *DGA* cycle and the secretaries of USDA and HHS affirm the list, the next task of collecting and evaluating data would begin. Original and existing systematic reviews, food pattern modeling, and descriptive data analyses would be conducted by federal methodologists (e.g., NEL staff, nutritional epidemiologists, respectively). TEPs would work with the federal teams as needed. Analyses ought to be conducted with the goal of providing final peer-reviewed results to the DGSAC when it first convenes (see Chapter 4). Some analyses are performed each cycle, such as identifying nutrients of concern, and could be produced before the DGPCG concludes its work, depending on data availability. If new data became available over the course of the *DGA* cycle that might lead to significant changes in results, it would be prudent to rerun analyses as needed.

Data Synthesis, Interpretation, and Integration

The final tasks in evaluating the body of evidence are data synthesis, interpretation, and integration, which would all be conducted by the DGSAC. This National Academies committee strongly believes that the DGSAC, as an independent arbiter of the state of the science, needs to be separated from data collection and evaluation to the greatest extent possible. While it will be necessary to work with the federal teams responsible for conducting systematic reviews, food pattern modeling, and descriptive data analyses, the role of the DGSAC needs to be clear, resulting in a different relationship than recent DGACs have had (see Chapter 4 for more details). By having more independence from the federal teams performing the analyses than in the current process, the DGSAC would be able to evaluate the evidence and develop conclusions without being able to unduly influence the process of data collection and evaluation.

The DGSAC would submit its final evaluation of the body of evidence to the secretaries of USDA and HHS in a scientific report. This scientific report ought to be open for public comment, similar to the public review of the current *DGAC Scientific Report*.

Update the *DGA*

Upon release of the DGSAC's scientific report, USDA and HHS would consider the DGSAC's conclusions in its update and review of the *DGA*, similar to what has been done with the 2005, 2010, and 2015 DGAC reports. Aside from selection of DGPCG, TEP, and DGSAC members, this final step of updating the *DGA* is the first place in the process policy makers should be involved in substantive decision making.

This National Academies committee believes that USDA and HHS should decide how the update is conducted, while making sure the process is transparent (see Chapter 5 for a full description and assessment of how USDA and HHS consider the *DGAC Scientific Report*).[5] For example, the federal writing team—the group that updates the *DGA* based on the *DGAC Scientific Report*—needs to adhere to explicit and transparent standards for developing evidence-based recommendations. Multiple sets of standards exist that could serve as models, with the understanding that the process for developing *DGA* recommendations does not follow typical guidelines development processes because the experts assessing the evidence do not write the guidelines and recommendations themselves.[6] As part of following these standards, it will be important to review the potential biases and conflicts of interest for writing team members, and ensure external reviewers represent a diverse set of viewpoints. As standards for the guidelines development process evolve, changes ought to be adopted by the federal writing team to keep the *DGA* process current with best practices in the field.

To enhance the integrity of the process, the *DGA Policy Report* should disclose what decisions were made about the DGSAC's conclusions and why any conclusions were not acted upon or modified.

Recommendation 2. The secretaries of USDA and HHS should provide the public with a clear explanation when the *DGA* omit or accept only parts of conclusions from the scientific report.

CONSIDERATION OF OPTIONS FOR IMPLEMENTATION

The proposed redesign model will not be easy to implement, but it is a necessary step to provide the process with agility and flexibility. This National Academies committee considered how the process redesign model could be implemented, while conforming to the National Nutrition Monitoring and Related Research Act and the Federal Advisory Committee Act; none of the recommended changes in this report would require a revision to either act.

This National Academies committee envisions the DGSAC as a federal advisory committee, like the DGAC has been. Constitution as a federal advisory committee would allow the DGSAC to provide con-

[5] The major steps include assembling a writing team of USDA and HHS staff, incorporating evidence, external peer review, and federal reviews and approvals.

[6] Organizations that have developed standards for clinical practice guidelines include the AGREE next steps consortium, the GRADE working group, the Guidelines International Network, the Institute of Medicine, and the World Health Organization (Brouwers et al., 2010; Guyatt et al., 2008; IOM, 2011; Oxman et al., 2006; Schünemann et al., 2012, 2013, 2014).

clusions to the secretaries of USDA and HHS based on the members' consensus. TEPs could be convened on an ad hoc basis by USDA and HHS. However, to allow for the DGPCG to operate continually under the constraint of the aforementioned laws, this National Academies committee has identified three options.

The first option is to establish the DGPCG as a federal advisory committee whose charter would be renewed every 2 years, the maximum length of time allowed under the Federal Advisory Committee Act. This option would allow the DGPCG to provide independent consensus-based recommendations to the secretaries in a transparent fashion. With the ability to be functionally continuous, the DGPCG would be able to help oversee efforts to monitor the literature. As a federal advisory committee, the DGPCG would recommend to the secretaries that its prioritized list of topics and questions be the set of topics reviewed by the DGSAC. USDA and HHS could informally share ownership of the process and operational costs, by each establishing a federal advisory committee (for example, USDA establish the DGPCG and HHS establish the DGSAC), thereby not overburdening any particular agency.[7] However, this option adds a degree of complexity to the current process that will require a number of handoffs between groups, necessitating coordination by USDA and HHS. Establishment of the DGPCG by a single agency could result in questions related to the independence of the DGPCG, as USDA's involvement in the *DGA* has been criticized in the past (Mozzaffarian, 2016). These concerns could be minimized if the checks in the process redesign model (e.g., more public comment periods, increased transparency at each step) were instituted.

A second option considered was establishing the DGPCG as a federal group consisting of both federal and nonfederal members, but not governed by the Federal Advisory Committee Act. As a federal group, the DGPCG could meet continually but could not issue consensus-based recommendations to the secretaries of USDA and HHS. This option could be seen as limiting transparency and jeopardizing the trustworthiness of the process based on the perception that USDA and HHS would have too much influence over the steps of monitoring new evidence and topic identification and prioritization. Other potential benefits and challenges regarding governance, funding, member composition and selection processes, and interactions with the DGSAC would depend in large part on

[7] Generally, only one agency can establish a discretionary, time-limited federal advisory committee so as to comply with federal restrictions related to the use of appropriated funds. Maintaining the current practice of rotating leadership and corresponding operational costs between the two agencies would require congressional authorization or presidential directive. This level of authority has not been needed for the current DGAC because it has not been acting in an ongoing manner.

how the federal group would be created and implemented. If this option was selected, creation of a federal group would need to be completed in a transparent manner.

A third option calls for a nongovernmental organization to convene the DGPCG. Term limits and other rules imposed by the Federal Advisory Committee Act would no longer apply and would also limit potential criticisms of USDA and HHS's roles. However, it is unclear whether advice from a nongovernmental organization would be as influential as options 1 and 2, particularly with respect to federal programs, or whether its processes would be transparent. It is also unlikely that a nongovernmental organization would have the funds and capacity to convene the DGPCG on its own. If this option were considered, organizations with the necessary breadth of expertise and experience would need to be identified.

Weighing the relative advantages and disadvantages of each option, this National Academies committee recognizes that no perfect option exists. Although option 1 adds layers of complexity with establishment of two federal advisory committees, it is the only option that features built-in mechanisms to ensure objectivity and transparency. Option 2 would potentially be the easiest to implement, but it is most likely to face criticism regarding its ability to perform the tasks of the DGPCG in a transparent and independent manner. Option 3 has great potential to ensure continuity and transparency, but it is dependent on numerous unknowable factors, most important of which is that an influential, nonpartisan organization with the necessary experience and expertise would need to be identified. Given these options, this National Academies committee believes establishing the DGPCG as a federal advisory committee to be the most likely option to yield a trustworthy, dependable evaluation of the science, without causing undue burden on any particular agency.

The presented model is one example of a new process that achieves the values and goals articulated in Chapter 2. This National Academies committee recognizes that the secretaries will need flexibility in implementing the proposed redesign, as there is no single best process to use. One reason for the need for flexibility is that a detailed exploration of the costs of the proposed redesign model could not be weighed in this report owing to a lack of information available regarding current resource use. This National Academies committee believes the operational costs would likely increase in the short term as a result of needing to set up and support the DGPCG, TEPs, and DGSAC. However, because the current DGAC tasks would be reallocated among the various groups, and over time the proposed process will likely simplify the number of questions being studied within each *DGA* cycle, it is this National Academies committee's judgment that costs may decrease in the long term. This National Academies committee believes the benefits and outcomes will justify any additional costs.

REFERENCES

Andrews, J. 2013. AHRQ methods for effective health care. In *Prioritization criteria methodology for future research needs proposals within the effective health care program: PiCMe-prioritization criteria methods.* Rockville, MD: Agency for Healthcare Research and Quality.

Brouwers, M., M. E. Kho, G. P. Browman, J. S. Burgers, F. Cluzeau, G. Feder, B. Fervers, I. D. Graham, J. Grimshaw, S. Hanna, P. Littlejohns, J. Makarski, and L. Zitzelsberger, for the AGREE Next Steps Consortium. 2010. AGREE II: Advancing guideline development, reporting and evaluation in healthcare. *Canadian Medical Association Journal* 182(18):E839-E842.

Guyatt, G. H., A. D. Oxman, R. Kunz, Y. Falck-Ytter, G. E. Vist, A. Liberati, and H. J. Schünemann. 2008. Going from evidence to recommendations. BMJ 336(7652):1049-1051.

HHS (U.S. Department of Health and Human Services). 2008. *The Secretary's Advisory Committee on National Health Promotion and Disease Prevention objectives for 2020: Phase I report recommendations for the framework and format of* Healthy People 2020. https://www.healthypeople.gov/sites/default/files/PhaseI_0.pdf (accessed July 14, 2017).

IOM (Institute of Medicine). 2011. *Clinical practice guidelines we can trust.* Washington, DC: The National Academies Press.

Mozzaffarian, D. 2016 (unpublished). *Comments presented at USDA* Dietary Guidelines for Americans *listening sessions.* Washington, DC, February 19, 2016.

Myers, E., A. J. McBroom, L. Shen, R. E. Posey, R. Gray, and G. D. Sanders. 2012. *Value-of-information analysis for patient-centered outcomes research prioritization.* Durham, NC: Duke Evidence-based Practice Center.

Oxman, A. D., A. Fretheim, and H. J. Schünemann. 2006. Improving the use of research evidence in guideline development: Introduction. *Health Research Policy and Systems* 4(1):12.

Schünemann, H. J., M. Woodhead, A. Anzueto, A. S. Buist, W. Macnee, K. F. Rabe, and J. Heffner. 2012. A guide to guidelines for professional societies and other developers of recommendations: Introduction to integrating and coordinating efforts in COPD guideline development. An official ATS/ERS workshop report. *Proceedings of the American Thoracic Society* 9(5):215-218.

Schünemann, H., J. Brožek, G. Guyatt, and A. Oxman, editors. 2013. *Handbook for grading the quality of evidence and the strength of recommendations using the GRADE approach.* The GRADE Working Group. http://gdt.guidelinedevelopment.org/app/handbook/handbook.html#h.33qgws879zw (accessed August 3, 2017).

Schünemann, H., W. Wiercioch, I. Etxeandia, M. Falavigna, N. Santesso, R. Mustafa, M. Ventresca, R. Brignardello-Petersen, K.-T. Laisaar, S. Kowalski, T. Baldeh, Y. Zhang, U. Raid, I. Neumann, S. L. Norris, J. Thornton, R. Harbour, S. Treweek, G. Guyatt, P. Alonso-Coello, M. Reinap, J. Brožek, A. Oxman, and E. A. Akl. 2014. Guidelines 2.0: Systematic development of a comprehensive checklist for a successful guideline enterprise. *Canadian Medical Association Journal* 186(3):E123-E142.

USDA (U.S. Department of Agriculture). 2017. *Pregnancy and birth to 24 months project.* https://www.cnpp.usda.gov/birthto24months (accessed January 8, 2017).

WHO (World Health Organization). 2017. *Normative work in nutrition at WHO: Priority setting for guideline development.* Geneva, Switzerland: World Health Organization.

4

Strengthening Analyses and Advancing Methods Used

The *Dietary Guidelines for Americans* (*DGA*)[1] must be based on the "preponderance of scientific and medical knowledge."[2] To achieve the goals of promoting health and reducing risk of chronic disease as proposed in Chapter 2, many types of inferential questions will need to be addressed, requiring that a wide range of information be considered to inform the *DGA*. To reach the most robust recommendations, the *DGA* also needs to be based on the highest standards of scientific evidence. Because scientific methods are continually evolving and new ones emerging, ensuring the scientific validity of the process to update the *DGA* will continue to depend on implementation of appropriate, validated, and standardized processes; adoption of strategic, efficient, and the most appropriate methods; and use of the most current high-quality data available. It will be critical to strengthen the data and analyses used in the *DGA*. Advancing the evidence underpinning the *DGA* will also require integrating newer methods that help better elucidate and represent the complex systems involved.

The *DGA* require the use of multiple sources of evidence. Data come from varying study designs, such as randomized trials and observational studies. These aggregate data, analyzed with the most current methodology, provide complementary information to answer different inferential questions and inform various parts of the evidence base. Properly evaluat-

[1] Refer to Chapter 1, Box 1-1, for an explanation of how the term *DGA* is used throughout this National Academies report.

[2] National Nutrition Monitoring and Related Research Act of 1990, Public Law 101-445, 101st Cong. (October 22, 1990), 7 U.S.C. 5341, 104 Stat. 1042–1044.

ing and calibrating results from a variety of data sources and methodological approaches are critical to understanding and interpreting the body of evidence to arrive at appropriate conclusions, as all study designs have innate limitations and can be susceptible to different types of bias. One key example is the complementary information derived from observational studies and randomized or controlled studies. If designed and conducted appropriately, randomized trials can control for confounders, allowing for causal relationships to be identified. Observational studies, because they do not use randomization to form comparison groups, can only establish association of effect and cannot be relied on to delineate mechanisms. However, given that many nutrition studies use observational designs and the populations and settings included more closely reflect the real world, these observational studies can provide other important insights that are complementary to the results of randomized trials. In addition, observational designs are employed when randomized trials cannot be conducted for reasons such as ethical concerns or logistical challenges. For instance, contextual information about the interface between foods and/or nutrients, as well as the interactions between diet and other factors can be derived from observational studies. Indeed, observational data have been used to provide important information in developing the *DGA*, such as data from surveys that inform findings related to disease prevalence and dietary intake patterns, among others. *DGA* recommendations will need to consider the results of multiple types of study designs.

The dual challenge faced in developing the *DGAC Scientific Report*, and subsequently the *DGA Policy Report*, is to properly assess the quality and interpret the results of studies available and to use them appropriately in drawing conclusions. The complexity of diet and health interactions necessitates the need for diverse types of analyses to inform strong and trustworthy conclusions. Taking the limitations of data and analyses into account in the collection, assessment, and decision-making process is crucial for building *DGA* that are based on the totality of scientific evidence and can be implemented.

This chapter first describes opportunities to strengthen the four types of analyses used by the 2015 Dietary Guidelines Advisory Committee (DGAC): (1) original Nutrition Evidence Library (NEL) systematic reviews; (2) existing systematic reviews, meta-analyses, and reports in the literature; (3) food pattern modeling analyses; and (4) descriptive data analyses (see Chapter 6 for a full description and assessment of each analysis and additional information on the strengths and limitations of data sources). Improving these types of analyses will help describe the systems that connect dietary intake with health outcomes of interest. This chapter then offers opportunities to adopt strategic, appropriate, and efficient methods to advance the review of the evidence.

STRENGTHENING EXISTING ANALYSES

Significant efforts have been made to standardize methods used to inform the *DGA* and to present the analyses transparently. For example, the NEL was introduced in 2010, and standard inclusion criteria for existing systematic reviews and meta-analyses were developed in 2015. In the past, DGACs have reviewed, synthesized, and drawn conclusions regarding the body of evidence on select topics. The evidence review process traditionally has encompassed a collection of multiple complementary types of analyses, as necessitated by the different types of questions reviewed by the DGAC. The 2015 DGAC based its conclusions on understanding the relationships between diet and health or disease outcomes, food patterns, and evidence related to prevalence of disease (see Table 6-1 for examples[3]).

This National Academies of Sciences, Engineering, and Medicine (the National Academies) committee envisions the work of the Dietary Guidelines Scientific Advisory Committee (DGSAC) to be focused on integrating results derived from multiple types of analyses (e.g., original systematic reviews; existing systematic reviews, meta-analyses, and reports; food pattern modeling; and descriptive data analyses) to develop conclusions about the totality of evidence relating diet and health (see Chapter 3 for additional details). One element of the process redesign model would be to create opportunities for analyses repeated in each *DGA* cycle to be prepared for review prior to the DGSAC's first meeting. Having standardized analyses (e.g., prevalence of a specific disease) conducted outside of the DGSAC's 2-year time frame of operation would allow the DGSAC to focus a greater proportion of its time synthesizing and interpreting the evidence and developing conclusions, as well as would facilitate comparisons between different cycles and over time. However, such analyses are contingent on the timing of the release of data from relevant surveys; availability of data may affect whether analyses can be completed before the DGSAC convenes. Approaches and methods that help better describe the systems and mechanisms involved also need to be used.

Systematic Reviews

This section describes opportunities to strengthen the conduct of NEL systematic reviews (de novo systematic reviews and updates) and the use of existing systematic reviews, meta-analyses, and reports.

---

[3] Table 6-1 includes three categories of questions (i.e., eating patterns, prevalence of disease, and relationships between diet and health) and provides examples from the *2015 DGAC Scientific Report*, as well as links the category of question to the type of analysis conducted in the 2005, 2010, 2015 DGACs (e.g., prevalence of disease questions, the 2015 DGAC conducted descriptive data analyses).

Nutrition Evidence Library Original Systematic Reviews

The NEL conducted systematic reviews to address questions from the 2015 DGAC regarding the relationship between diet and health. While these important questions provided key inputs into the *DGA*, and will continue to do so, they are difficult to answer and require a strong body of evidence. The methods for conducting systematic reviews are crucial for developing trustworthy *DGA*. This National Academies committee assessed the NEL systematic review process, identifying several opportunities to advance and align the NEL protocol with existing best practices for systematic reviews.

As described in Chapter 6, the NEL original systematic review process to inform the *2010* and *2015 DGAC Scientific Reports* has been facilitated by NEL staff, but staff relied heavily on input from the DGAC at each step to guide the process (see Box 4-1). However, standards for conducting systematic reviews and guidelines call for the clear delineation of roles in order to minimize the introduction of bias and allow for an objective, evidence-based review. Those who synthesize and interpret the evidence and formulate conclusions ought *not* to be leading the development of the systematic review protocol and selection of studies (e.g., inclusion/exclusion criteria) (AHRQ, 2014; Balshem et al., 2011; Guyatt et al., 2011). Drawing on the appropriate methodological and domain expertise in the systematic review process allows for robust outcomes while also maximizing time and resources for both NEL staff and outside expertise (e.g., a technical expert panel). As proposed in the process redesign model in Chapter 3, the NEL ought to focus on the following:

- Planning and conducting systematic reviews;
- Adhering to the specified protocol, including assisting in the development of systematic review questions;
- Conducting the literature search and screening and selecting articles;
- Abstracting data; and
- Conducting a risk of bias assessment[4] in individual studies.

A technical expert panel (TEP) would provide supplemental domain and methodological expertise to the NEL at various steps as needed during the development of systematic reviews. The DGSAC's role would be focused primarily on synthesizing the results of multiple systematic

[4] A risk of bias assessment refers to evaluating the potential of bias in an individual study or collection of studies. Several published protocols are available for conducting a risk of bias assessment (AHRQ, 2014; Higgins and Green, 2011; IOM, 2011; Schünemann et al., 2013). The NEL process for conducting a risk of bias assessment is described in Chapter 6.

BOX 4-1
NEL Systematic Review Steps

Step 1: Topic identification and systematic review question development

- Identify topics
- Develop questions
- Prioritize questions
- Develop analytic framework

Step 2: Literature search, screening, and selection

- Refine inclusion/exclusion criteria
- Develop search strategy
- Screen and select studies
- Determine inclusion of existing systematic reviews/meta-analyses/reports

Step 3: Data extraction and risk of bias assessment

- Extract data
- Assess risk of bias

Step 4: Evidence description and synthesis

- Synthesize and evaluate evidence
- Draft evidence description and synthesis

Step 5: Conclusion statement development and evidence grading

- Draft conclusion statement
- Grade body of evidence/conclusion statement

Step 6: Identification of research recommendations

SOURCE: USDA/HHS, 2016.

reviews and interpreting the body of evidence (see Box 4-2 for a description of terms). If needed, the NEL could assist the DGSAC in its synthesis of systematic review results given its familiarity with the primary studies. However, the interpretation of the body of evidence would be left solely to the DGSAC.

To be transparent, the NEL would need to make a number of its steps publicly available. These steps include the systematic review protocol, a rationale for each question being asked, inclusion and exclusion criteria, and reasons for why an article was or was not included in the review.

BOX 4-2
Terminology Used Describing the Various Steps Related to Evaluating Systematic Reviews

Synthesis refers to the process of combining data from multiple sources. This can be objective or subjective depending on the type of data, as it includes both the (1) evaluation of the results across multiple studies in a systematic review (e.g., the qualitative or quantitative analysis of study results) and (2) the evaluation of multiple components within a single study (e.g., the combination of correlated outcomes in a single study).

Interpretation refers to the subjective process of building on synthesis results to develop the DGSAC's conclusions about a single study, multiple studies, or systematic reviews (e.g., interpretation of a risk of bias assessment for an individual study; interpretation of heterogeneity across multiple studies to decide whether to combine studies; interpretation of whether or not there is a strong relationship between diet and cardiovascular disease based on a systematic review).

Integration in this report is used to mean combining the results of systematic reviews, food pattern modeling, descriptive data analysis, and any other types of evidence to develop the DGSAC's conclusions on the total body of evidence for the *DGA*.

Additionally, an independent, external peer-review process for NEL systematic reviews will be critical to help increase the credibility of the systematic reviews. Peer review also provides opportunities to identify and correct any outstanding errors in the systematic review in advance of consideration by the DGSAC. To obtain an objective assessment, peer reviewers would ideally not have been involved with other steps of the process as members of the NEL or DGSAC. TEP members would only be involved as one of many peer reviewers, and not in a leading role. Although the NEL could facilitate the peer-review process, this National Academies committee suggests that the NEL explore existing infrastructures, such as collaborating with nutrition-focused scientific journals, to facilitate implementation of a peer-review process. This would reduce the need for the NEL to develop an infrastructure to support a peer review for individual systematic reviews. Collaborating with a peer-reviewed journal may also have the additional benefit of increasing the likelihood of publication of the systematic review. It would not be necessary for the systematic review to be published prior to consideration by the DGSAC due to time constraints. The NEL staff ought to consider publishing systematic reviews in peer-reviewed journals as appropriate. One example of this type of relationship is exemplified by collaborations that the Agency for Healthcare Research and Quality (AHRQ) Evidence-based Practice Centers Program has with peer-reviewed journals to conduct reviews and publish systematic reviews. All NEL systematic reviews should be peer reviewed to the extent possible. If time does not allow for the NEL to fully integrate peer-review comments into a revised systematic review, an alternative would be to share the original draft along with peer-review comments to the DGSAC for consideration as it synthesizes results and interprets the body of evidence.

Recommendation 3. The secretary of USDA should clearly separate the roles of USDA Nutrition Evidence Library (NEL) staff and the Dietary Guidelines Scientific Advisory Committee (DGSAC) such that

a. The NEL staff plan and conduct systematic reviews with input from technical expert panels, perform risk of bias assessment of individual studies, and assist the DGSAC as needed.

b. The NEL systematic reviews are externally peer reviewed prior to being made available for use by the DGSAC.

c. The DGSAC synthesizes and interprets the results of systematic reviews and draws conclusions about the entire body of evidence.

Several best practices for systematic reviews have evolved and continue to be improved since the NEL systematic review protocol was developed. For the NEL to remain current and to continue to produce systematic reviews of the highest quality, this National Academies committee offers recommendations for the NEL to maintain state-of-the-art systematic review methods. Opportunities for collaboration and learning from other organizations should be leveraged, as well as training and support for NEL staff to actively engage in maintaining an up-to-date systematic review protocol. By instituting ongoing training and collaboration and supportive methodological infrastructure to cultivate systematic review practitioners with a nutrition focus, the NEL has the opportunity to become a leading evidence source for the nutrition community. Of note, some of the best practices identified by this National Academies committee—for example, the delineation of roles and the introduction of a TEP in developing systematic review questions—have already been integrated into the NEL process for conducting systematic reviews outside of the DGAC (see Chapter 6 for a description of the non-DGAC NEL process[5]). The systematic review pro-

[5] The non-DGAC NEL process parallels the NEL process in many regards. The fundamental difference is that in the DGAC process, decisions are made by the DGAC with support

tocol used to conduct systematic reviews ought to reflect best practices to the extent feasible.

An explicit evaluation of how each step of the NEL protocol was *implemented* in previous *DGA* cycles was outside of this National Academies committee's charge. However, critics have offered serious concerns that the implementation of the NEL protocol needs improvement (Heimowitz, 2016; Mozzaffarian, 2016; Trumbo, 2017; Willett, 2016). One possible improvement would be to invite systematic review experts to periodically assess the NEL process, as well as to learn from other leading organizations (e.g., AHRQ, Cochrane). Such relationships would be beneficial in particularly challenging steps of systematic reviews (e.g., implementation of grading criteria,[6] evaluation of evidence). For example, AHRQ has several methods working groups that periodically review and update methods. While AHRQ and Cochrane have traditionally focused on conducting nonnutrition systematic reviews, there are enough overlaps in the process with nutrition systematic reviews that the NEL could benefit from participation in these forums. Furthermore, AHRQ and Cochrane at times also perform nutrition reviews, which could facilitate two-way collaboration between the NEL and other organizations.

Another opportunity for collaboration and alignment with best practices is in synthesizing and interpreting the body of evidence. These are subjective processes and require experience and expertise. As such, a standard and up-to-date approach is necessary to account for the strengths and the limitations of included studies, as well as to formulate evidence-based conclusions. In reviewing the current NEL process, this National Academies committee identified three opportunities for improvement:

1. Use specific criteria/limit subjective criteria (e.g., explicit definition of a "large, high-quality, and/or consistent body of evidence")
2. Use quantitative confidence intervals (e.g., specific numeric confidence intervals in "high level of certainty")
3. Define explicit mechanisms for moving study grades up or down (e.g., explicit definition of "methodological or generalizability concerns")

---

by the NEL in accordance with the Federal Advisory Committee Act. In contrast, in the non-DGAC NEL process, the NEL makes key decisions relating to systematic review methodology and relies on a technical expert collaborative for domain expertise. The non-DGAC NEL process also differs from the DGAC NEL process with respect to tools used for risk of bias assessment and evaluating the strength of a body of evidence.

[6] Grading refers to evaluating a body of evidence in a systematic review. Several published protocols are available for evaluating a body of evidence according to specific criteria (AHRQ, 2014; Higgins and Green, 2011; IOM, 2011; Schünemann et al., 2013). The NEL criteria for grading are described in Chapter 6.

Conduct of original systematic reviews will need to be transparent and follow state-of-the-art methods, such as the GRADE approach and the AHRQ Evidence-based Practice Centers Program approach. However, this National Academies committee believes the NEL and DGSAC need to have the flexibility to align with appropriate standards or methods and does not recommend that any one standard be adopted, which may be subject to change and evolve over time. In assessing the overall evidence review process, this National Academies committee explored the options for conducting systematic reviews within the NEL, as well as options outside the NEL, such as contracting out a limited number of systematic reviews to be performed by external groups. However, there are advantages of a dedicated team conducting systematic reviews like the NEL, rather than contracting to outside groups. A dedicated in-house team has domain knowledge and institutional memories that can learn from past experiences. Compared with contracting with external sources, a dedicated team would likely be able to respond in a more nimble and timely manner to requests for systematic reviews.

Recommendation 4. The secretary of USDA should ensure all Nutrition Evidence Library (NEL) systematic reviews align with best practices by

a. Enabling ongoing training of the NEL staff,
b. Enabling engagement with and learning from external groups on the forefront of systematic review methods,
c. Inviting external systematic review experts to periodically evaluate the NEL's methods, and
d. Investing in technological infrastructure.

Updating Systematic Reviews

In alignment with the need to increase adaptability and flexibility as outlined in Chapter 2, ongoing surveillance of the literature on any given topic is necessary to ensure that systematic reviews are up to date while maximizing use of resources. Determining when systematic reviews should be updated depends on a number of signals. In conducting a systematic review, the authors may assign the review a length of time for which the conclusions are expected to be relevant, or in other words, an "expiration date." This may be determined based on the topic, known current research, expectations of future research, and the strength of the evidence, and ensures systematic reviews reflect the most current body of literature. After that time frame, to ensure conclusions remain relevant, reviews ought to be continually monitored and updated as needed based on new evidence or shifting priorities and questions. This National Academies committee envisions the ongoing surveillance and consideration for updating systematic reviews to be an activity of the NEL staff with input from the DGPCG.

Once a topic has been selected for the DGSAC to review, surveillance efforts ought to identify relevant existing systematic reviews. Upon identification, these existing systematic reviews would need to be evaluated for their timeliness and methodological quality. Updates may be needed, such as an updated search of the literature to identify possible new studies, a new search strategy to incorporate new questions, or additional analyses to be performed.

Updates of systematic reviews should be performed purposefully with the goal of answering a specific question. Revisions can be made on one's own systematic reviews or those produced by others. Updating one's own systematic reviews may be easier if all the data are standardized in their collection and archival. To ensure efficiency, data used in a previous systematic review will need to be readily available in a form that could be reused or could have new data elements added to it.

Existing Systematic Reviews

For the 2015 DGAC, efforts were made to use the existing literature to supplement or replace the need for an original review when a topic or question was reviewed that had already been addressed in existing systematic reviews, meta-analyses, and reports from leading organizations. The 2015 DGAC established a set of quality criteria that existing systematic reviews, meta-analyses, and reports needed to meet in order to be incorporated into the evidence base, including the relevance of the existing systematic review to the question of interest, the quality of the systematic review, the timeliness, and the reference overlap if multiple existing systematic reviews or meta-analyses were used for the same question (see Chapter 6 for a detailed description of how these criteria were implemented by the 2015 DGAC). No specific criteria were used by the NEL to evaluate existing reports.

Overall, this National Academies committee believes that using existing high-quality systematic reviews whenever possible maximizes limited time and resources and reduces duplication of efforts. However, it is important to recognize that existing systematic reviews may not use the same inclusion and exclusion criteria, may be out of date, or may have different outcomes (Smith et al., 2011; Whitlock et al., 2008). As a result, using existing systematic reviews may be more time and resource intensive than conducting de novo systematic reviews. The criteria upon which to evaluate the quality of existing systematic reviews currently outlined by the NEL have generally been appropriate for determining relevance and inclusion or exclusion, but the criteria will need to be updated to keep pace with advances in systematic review methods, such as changes to AMSTAR and the Risk of Bias in Systematic Review tool (AMSTAR, 2016; Shea and Henry, 2016; Whiting et al., 2016).

Regardless of the type of systematic review being conducted or for whom (both NEL DGAC and non-DGAC systematic reviews), the NEL ought to follow a single set of standards, which needs to be transparent and of the highest quality. As systematic review methods evolve, the process to update the *DGA* will need to follow. For example, it is important to recognize that the quality, and thus the usefulness, of systematic reviews are dependent on the rigor of the original data. It will be up to the DGSAC and the DGPCG to determine how to develop conclusions based on low-quality data, as well as to identify areas where more research is needed to strengthen the evidence base. The NEL will need to adopt advances in systematic review methods to address the limitations related to low-quality data. Reproducibility is another methodological issue that will continue to be a problem in the future. Systematic review methods will continue to evolve and it will be important for the NEL and DGSAC to stay abreast of the literature in order to best adapt the methods used in the *DGA* process. Another example of an improvement in systematic review methods is the development of core outcome sets that could facilitate synthesis and comparison of systematic reviews, which could be part of the DGPCG strategic planning role (Clarke and Williamson, 2016; COMET Initiative, 2017). Additionally, systematic reviews have traditionally relied on summary results, or averages across all subjects in a study, reported in publications. With the advent of the requirement that trials be registered, the increase in patient registries, and the overall move toward open science, individual patient-level data will become more commonly available. Enhanced information can be extracted from individual patient-level data as compared to summary data. These improvements in systematic review methods will likely affect the analyses underlying the *DGA*.

Food Pattern Modeling

Food pattern modeling serves the important function of showing examples of ways individual diets can both meet energy (caloric) constraints and support intake of necessary nutrients at sufficient levels to promote health and prevent disease. The process to develop food patterns, as well as a number of important assumptions inherent in the process, is discussed in detail in Chapter 6. Box 4-3 lists the primary steps in food pattern modeling. Previous DGACs incorporated food pattern modeling in their reviews of the evidence, based on current food consumption

BOX 4-3
Food Pattern Modeling Steps

1. Establish energy levels
2. Establish nutrient goals
3. Establish food groups
4. Develop food groups composites and nutrient profiles
5. Model inputs and constraints

patterns and recommended nutrient intakes. In addition to translating nutrient requirements into food combinations, the models were also used to estimate how well various combinations of foods eaten on a daily or a weekly basis, called "eating patterns," met Dietary Reference Intakes and recommendations in the *DGA* to promote health and prevent disease. Overall, this National Academies committee found food pattern modeling to be a useful exercise to elucidate relationships among food group nutrient profiles, nutrient goals, and energy constraints that helped inform decision making by the DGAC and the federal *DGA* writing team.

Diet constitutes an extremely complex system of exposure that is known to influence health, and these modeling exercises can help make sense of that complex system. Food pattern modeling has traditionally focused on representing the overall population through use of population average energy and nutrient requirements, typical food choices, and a traditional American diet set of food groups. However, the heterogeneity of the population is largely not accounted for, such as the distribution of requirements for energy and all nutrients, widely varying food choices by numerous demographic factors, and some food groups not being consumed by all Americans. Accordingly, food pattern models will be more useful as methods are strengthened to adapt to new areas of science, a better appreciation of the systems involved is formed, more systems science methods become available, and technology becomes increasingly more sophisticated. Food pattern modeling has employed set estimates for various inputs, a process known as deterministic modeling. Stochastic systems modeling, which more extensively and specifically accounts for variability and uncertainty, would be preferable, because making dietary recommendations as transparent, applicable, and robust as possible increases their ability to account for the complex systems involved and the variabilities in food composition and consumption. Simulation systems modeling is a type of stochastic modeling that could result in more real-life answers. Sensitivity analyses can then explore the effect of systematically varying different parameters.

A greater understanding of the variability in the estimates could readily be applied in two areas. The first is the range of nutrient values associated with each set of food group recommendations. All the nutrient profiles and the total nutrients associated with each pattern are dependent on the quality of the food composition data used to derive the estimates. For this purpose, USDA uses its own databases, which represent the nutrition field standard. However, it uses only the average composition values, rather than incorporating the information on variability surrounding the values that could enhance confidence in the adequacy of the patterns.

A second area where sensitivity analyses might be applied is in varying combinations of recommendations to achieve nutrient targets. This includes expansion of food patterns to show multiple ways to achieve targets. To some degree, the Mediterranean and vegetarian patterns reflect this concept, but further deviations from the American norm could be explored. For example, many Asian groups consume little to no dairy foods and use rice as a staple grain rather than wheat.

Because the complexity of the modeling may increase many fold with such adaptations, a stepwise approach toward additional layers of intricacy is warranted to see how each change affects the results. At the same time, development of system models can be facilitated by incorporating newer, more powerful, and more efficient computational techniques such as automated algorithms, rather than the current iterative approach that could become unwieldy, given the breadth of foods to be considered as inputs into the models. As nutritional recommendations are likely to become more personalized in the future, the adjustments to food pattern modeling will need to follow suit. For example, appropriate energy intake levels might be tailored according to whether a person is at, over, or below ideal weight, and food intolerances such as allergies could be accounted for in building patterns. As with any modeling, it will be important to include an evaluation of the certainty regarding the input parameters in future approaches.

Even using the relatively limited deterministic approach, food pattern modeling reveals the very small allowance for discretionary calories relative to population intakes of energy from added sugars, solid fats, and alcohol. This revelation is critically important, and yet understanding by the public of how the resulting patterns should be interpreted and followed seems to be lacking, as evidenced by the discordance between recommendations and usual intakes (Krebs-Smith et al., 2010; NCI, 2015). Furthermore, the national food supply is not consistent with these patterns; for example, the mix of foods entering retail distribution channels does not represent the balance among fruits, vegetables, whole grains, dairy, protein foods, and empty calories as recommended by federal guidance (Miller et al., 2015). Results and implications of food pattern modeling exercises should be evaluated for how well they are implemented across the food supply chain.

In summary, this National Academies committee determined that food pattern modeling, as currently conducted, answers an important but narrow set of questions with appropriate methodologies. However, more key questions involving different assumptions could be addressed with a more expansive use of modeling and system science. Advancing the methods used in food pattern modeling to account for the complex systems and associated pathways and variability in American diets would strengthen the accuracy of outcomes and better account for the variability in food patterns and their resulting impact to support health and prevent disease. These advancements would offer important insights into the range of nutrients and the varying combinations of "allowable" foods to stay within dietary guidelines, providing flexibility in food and taste preferences, cultural norms, and other individual factors. In addition, complex systems models more accurately represent the dynamic nature of food and eating patterns, and they can be adapted to changing diets and population needs over time, as well as reflect future advancements in methods. It will also be critical for researchers to translate findings from these models for the general population.

Recommendation 5. The secretaries of USDA and HHS should enhance food pattern modeling to better reflect the complex interactions involved, variability in intakes, and range of possible healthful diets.

Descriptive Data Analyses

Descriptive data analyses provide key insights to understanding the context and landscape of dietary patterns and population health and disease, including both current intakes and prevalence of disease. Data analyses to inform the 2015 DGAC's review of the evidence constituted examinations of primary data sources to answer descriptive questions about the overall population and population subgroups, such as "What are current consumption patterns of nutrients from foods and beverages by the U.S. population?" (for a full list of questions, see Appendix C). For dietary intakes, the DGAC relied primarily on the dietary portion of What We Eat in America (WWEIA) of the National Health and Nutrition Examination Survey (NHANES), which uses self-reported dietary intake data through the 24-hour dietary recall method. The 2015 DGAC also used other selected data sources (see Table 6-5 for a summary of data sources used in the *Scientific Report of the 2015*

DGAC).[7] In the past, the data analyses were initiated concurrently with the convening of the DGAC. However, data analyses could be made more efficient by identifying questions earlier and having available data sooner, allowing for select data analyses to be performed before the first meeting of the DGSAC. In most instances, the data sources and analyses used by the 2015 DGAC addressed the questions it posed. It would be helpful for data analyses to be standardized to the extent possible to allow for direct comparisons of results over time. This National Academies committee also found that the availability of data can limit the scope of the data analyses, and the expansion of data collection efforts and advancement of methods could lead to improvements in the understanding of population health and disease prevalence and trends, particularly for population subgroups.

One area that would be particularly important to standardize, both within and across DGSAC cycles, is identification of nutrients of concern—an evaluation of the prevalence of nutrient inadequacies and excesses in the U.S. population and select population groups and associated health implications (see Chapter 7 for additional discussion). Identification of nutrients of concern would allow the DGSAC to focus on select nutrients that, if either increased or decreased compared to current intake levels, could affect population health. Nutrients of concern also can drive subsequent implementation and education efforts, and they have also been used as food sector reformulations to vary nutrient levels in products. The analytic approach to determining the proportion of the population with inadequate intakes or at risk of adverse effects owing to excess consumption has been relatively comparable across the past three editions of the *DGAC Scientific Report*. However, the interpretation and application of those quantitative assessments has differed across the various cycles. Differences include the thresholds used to define a nutrient as being of concern, and the degree to which biochemical and chronic disease-related data were available and used to justify the designation (see Chapter 7 for additional details). As validated biomarkers that are surrogate end points of chronic disease become available, it will be important to understand how biomarker research can be included into the *DGA* evidence review process.

An adoption of a more consistent approach to designating nutrients of concern in a DGAC conclusion would benefit practitioners, consumers, and the food sector. Such an approach would standardize the quantita-

---

[7] Other data sources used for information on health conditions and trends and disease prevalence were the American Heart Association statistics, the National Health Interview Survey, the SEARCH for Diabetes in Youth study, and the National Cancer Institute's Surveillance, Epidemiology, and End Results Program. The USDA-ARS National Nutrient Database for Standard Reference, Release 27 was used for food composition data.

tive threshold of inadequacy or excess and the integration of other supporting evidence to identify a nutrient of concern. As described in the process redesign model in Chapter 3, development of data inputs ought to be independent from the DGSAC, similar to the delineated roles of the DGSAC and the NEL for systematic reviews.

Recommendation 6. The secretaries of USDA and HHS should standardize the methods and criteria for establishing nutrients of concern.

A standard approach to identifying diet-related chronic disease for inclusion in the *DGA* would also be helpful. Knowing which chronic diseases are affected by diet, as well as what diets have been linked with decreasing or increasing risk of development of chronic disease, are integral to producing guidelines that can reduce the risk of chronic disease. However, the science to explain these relationships needs further research in order to establish the mechanisms underlying diet and health.

To conclude, descriptive data analyses can be useful in guiding the conclusions of the DGSAC. Common analyses can be performed in each cycle to inform key decisions. Consistent use of standardized approaches to descriptive data analyses, including prevalence in the population beyond which a nutrient is considered of concern, would facilitate comparisons between different cycles and over time. Descriptive data analyses could also benefit from peer review if applicable. Although flexibility can allow for adaptations and responses to changes for areas in which evidence and methodologies are rapidly emerging, applying a standardized approach across *DGA* cycles would allow for a more direct comparison of evidence across reports. It would be valuable, as a first step, to document all the descriptive data analyses commonly used across previous DGACs.

Quality of Dietary Data Across All Evidence Types

It is important that the data informing the *DGSAC Scientific Report* are generated using validated and appropriate methods. The analysis and interpretation of the data also need to be consistent with best practices. Box 4-4 discusses several resources for improving the quality of self-reported dietary intake data.[8] In addition to providing a transparent con-

[8] Self-report dietary intake data are central to the development of dietary guidelines. Measurement error is a substantial limitation of self-report dietary intake data, and can lead to various degrees of bias based on the method of collecting self-report dietary intake data (NCI, 2017). Several methods exist to address the effects of measurement error. See Chapter 6 for an explanation of the types of measurement error and implications for appropriate use of self-report dietary intake data.

BOX 4-4
Collecting and Using Self-Reported Dietary Intake Data

It is important for researchers to adopt current best practices for data collection, data analyses, and reporting of their studies. Detailed resources are available to facilitate analysis and interpretation of self-reported data to align with best practices in the field. For example, the National Cancer Institute's *Dietary Assessment Primer* provides guidance to researchers on how to use the major dietary assessment instruments alone or in combination to address descriptive, epidemiological, and intervention-related questions (NCI, 2017). The *Primer* also provides extensive background on measurement error and validation. The STrengthening Reporting of OBservational Epidemiology (STROBE-nut) checklist is a tool to help researchers improve the quality of reporting nutrition studies. This tool was developed via a systematic process by a multidisciplinary team and provides 24 guidelines on best practices for adding clarity to studies regarding a range of issues including dietary assessment methods, measurement error adjustments, validity testing, and statistical methods (Lachat et al., 2016).

Biomarkers are also increasingly being recognized as an important adjunct in measuring dietary intakes because they provide more objective data. Biomarkers that relate to dietary intake can be obtained from samples of blood, urine, or tissues, or with noninvasive testing of body tissues, such as carotenoid content measured optically. Currently these are only available for a subset of nutrients and bioactive compounds of interest in nutrition. Recovery biomarkers are of greatest value because they are not subject to homeostasis or interindividual differences in metabolism and provide objective unbiased measures of absolute intake. The limited number of recovery biomarkers includes doubly labeled water, which reflects energy expenditure and therefore energy intake in weight stable individuals, and urinary nitrogen, sodium, and potassium, which reflect dietary protein, sodium, and potassium, respectively. Concentration biomarkers comprise a slightly larger set, but they are subject to interindividual differences in metabolism; that is, they exhibit their own form of measurement error regarding dietary intake. These can be used in conjunction with self-report data and statistical modeling as an indirect measure of intake. The identification of additional biomarkers and prediction equations could improve the accuracy of dietary data.

Even if biomarkers could be identified for every food and nutrient of interest, they could not replace self-reported dietary intake data, especially dietary recalls and records because dietary intake data provide complementary, contextual information about timing and place of meals, foods eaten in combination, and even the foods themselves that biomarkers cannot differentiate. Biomarkers cannot distinguish, for example, a tomato eaten as part of a salad from a tomato eaten as part of a hamburger sandwich or a tomato eaten as part of ketchup. Such differences in consumption may be relevant to health, for example, if they influence energy intake and energy balance. Furthermore, self-reports reflect food intakes in terms that are salient to the individual, such as pizza and ice cream, rather than the more abstract notions of nutrients or other food constituents. Consequently, such information is critical for back-translating information about diet/health relationships in terms the population can understand.

continued

BOX 4-4 Continued

No perfect measure of diet exists, principally because diet is such a complex, multidimensional, and dynamic exposure. Ongoing scientific controversy highlights the diversity of scientific opinions on the usefulness of the more biased methodologies. Some critics have questioned the use of self-reported intake methods entirely (Dhurandhar et al., 2015). Others have proposed opportunities to recognize the limitations of self-reported data and ensure they are properly accounted for in both the analysis and interpretation of the data (Subar et al., 2015). Data can provide useful information on which to guide dietary choices if appropriate methods are chosen, and measurement error and other limitations are recognized and reported appropriately.

sideration of the quality of food intake data, future data analyses could be made more efficient by identifying questions earlier and having available data sooner, allowing for select data analyses to be performed before the first meeting of the DGSAC. It would also be helpful for selection of data and data analyses to be standardized using best practices to the extent possible to allow for direct comparisons of results over time.

ADVANCING METHODS USED

The types of questions asked by recent DGACs have been limited by the available evidence, data, and methods. Strengthening the data available and the statistical and epidemiologic analyses conducted will enhance important insights regarding factors in the diet–health relationship. These approaches, however, are not designed to understand how strings of actions, reactions, and new actions among multiple health-relevant sectors and diet may affect an overall system outcome such as weight and chronic disease occurrence. These insights are the domain of complex systems science with methods such as systems dynamics, agent-based modeling, and network modeling (El-Sayed and Galea, 2017; Sterman, 2006). Incorporating systems science approaches to data and evidence assessment in the *DGA* process can extend the value provided by better data and traditional analytical methods.

Developments in knowledge and data, as well as computing systems and computational methods and capabilities, now present opportunities to approach relationships in diet and health with an appreciation for the complexity that exists in the real world. As discussed in Chapter 2, this National Academies committee believes that adding complex systems approaches to current analytical approaches can advance the understanding of complex interrelated factors at play in both population and individual health. Systems approaches have been used successfully in addressing many public health challenges (see Box 4-5 for examples).

Specific examples of systems mapping and modeling linking nutrition and health are limited (Lee et al., 2017b). Integrating systems approaches into the field of nutrition will require the same bold experimentation with systems science methods that was undertaken in other domains when no evidence of its value for their specific application existed. This is a cultural shift. Currently, nutrition research, and thus the *DGA* process, begins with the available data and looks for trends in those data. The cultural shift would involve researchers beginning with a systems map and model, which represent the relationships and potential mechanisms involved, and then using the model to help prioritize and guide the collection and analysis of data. Developing and enhancing the maps and models is an essential and iterative process.

Previous DGACs have recognized the potential value and discussed the need to move toward use of systems approaches. The 2015 DGAC integrated a theoretical model that accounted for the multidimensional relationship and multiple factors influencing both dietary intake and health (see Figure 7-1 for the 2015 DGAC conceptual map). It is now time to translate this theoretical systems discussion into an actual application to the *DGA* process, including building systems maps and integrating systems models as an expanded analytic framework for the evidence review. Systems thinking, when fully integrated into the *DGA* process and supported with systems mapping and modeling, has the potential to influence the *DGA* recommendations based on an expanded knowledge of the diet–health relationships of interest, inform the translation of the guidelines to maximize impact, and identify relevant connections across stakeholders. Systems maps, by highlighting areas of stronger and weaker evidence, can also help to prioritize subsequent research and data collection needs. Within the *DGA* process, there would be a dynamic, interdependent relationship between the systems maps, models, data, questions of interest, and recommendations for the *DGA* and future directions. For example, building a systems map could inform key topic and question development. The DGSAC's review of the evidence could provide data inputs in the development of a systems model. Additionally, the outputs of the systems maps and models could provide important inputs into the *DGA*.

It is important to understand the range of different types of modeling approaches and how they differ in their strengths and weaknesses and ability to represent the interactions and mechanisms involved. On one end of the spectrum are "deterministic" statistical modeling and epidemiological approaches that take existing datasets and help identify associations and trends and make predictions, but do not necessarily elu-

BOX 4-5
Examples of How Systems Approaches Have Been Applied in Other Fields

Childhood Body Mass Index and Physical Activity

An example of using a systems model to better understand and represent the pathway between a type of behavior and health outcomes is physical activity and weight during childhood (Lee et al., 2017a). For this model, researchers first mapped out the relationship between increasing a child's physical activity and the child's weight and then developed a computational model that could simulate this relationship (i.e., how increasing physical activity may then decrease weight and body mass index [BMI]). The relationship between BMI during childhood and BMI during adulthood was mapped. A third step was mapping out the relationship between adult BMI and the risk of different major chronic diseases such as diabetes, heart disease, cerebrovascular disease, and cancer. The final step of the mapping was drawing the relationships between these diseases and health outcomes such as myocardial infarction, stroke, quality of life, and life expectancy. Once the mapping was completed, the next phase was converting this map into a dynamic computational model that could then simulate all of these relationships and processes over time. This then allowed experiments such as determining what would happen if the physical activity of a child was increased. How would this affect various relevant health outcomes?

Policy Impact Assessment in Cardiovascular Health Using Systems Science

Systems models have shown how different clinical and biometric factors and social determinants of health interact to influence cardiovascular health. For example, a systems model developed by Homer et al. (2008) provides a policy framework for assessing impacts on cardiovascular risk, accounting for lifestyle and behavioral, social, and environmental conditions. Local contextual factors such as food access and availability, eating patterns and physical activity options, socioeconomic conditions, environmental policies, and support service options can have important influences on cardiovascular risk and are captured in the model. Also included in the systems model are health services utilization and individual factors such as intake of fruits and vegetables, net calories, physical activity, and stress. The model shows that, together, local context; utilization of services; and nutrition, physical activity, and stress all affect cardiovascular disease risk factor

cidate and represent the actual mechanisms involved. Examples include traditional epidemiological studies that can reveal patterns and associations and attempt to control for confounding factors, such as selection and observation biases. Randomized or controlled trials may be able to answer specific efficacy questions but occur in a nonreal-world, controlled setting and thus do not represent all or even most of the interactions and mechanisms that are operative in the real world (i.e., a given complex prevalence and control. Simulation experiments using the model provided insights into the dynamic interactions among the various components and risk factors, as well as their resulting impact on the prevalence rates of cardiovascular disease and the costs of treating versus preventing cardiovascular events. The model can also be used to inform policy decisions, such as how increasing access to affordable and healthful foods and other hypothetical interventions can reduce cardiovascular risk and adverse events.

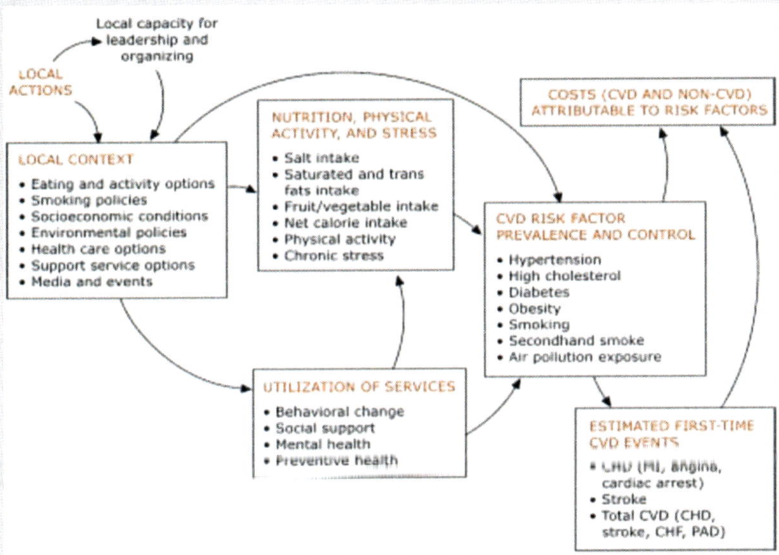

A policy framework for cardiovascular risk.
NOTE: CHD = coronary heart disease; CHF = congestive heart failure; CVD = cardiovascular disease; MI = myocardial infarction; PAD = peripheral arterial disease.
SOURCE: Homer et al., 2008.

system). By contrast, systems modeling is essentially a "nondeterministic" approach that attempts to simulate real-world heterogeneity and the relationships and array of mechanisms that affect the relationship between diet and health. By trying to build a representation of a system, the system overall can be better understood, as well as the dependencies and potential effects of the various system components on a given outcome or risk.

Figure 4-1 shows that implementation of systems approaches for the

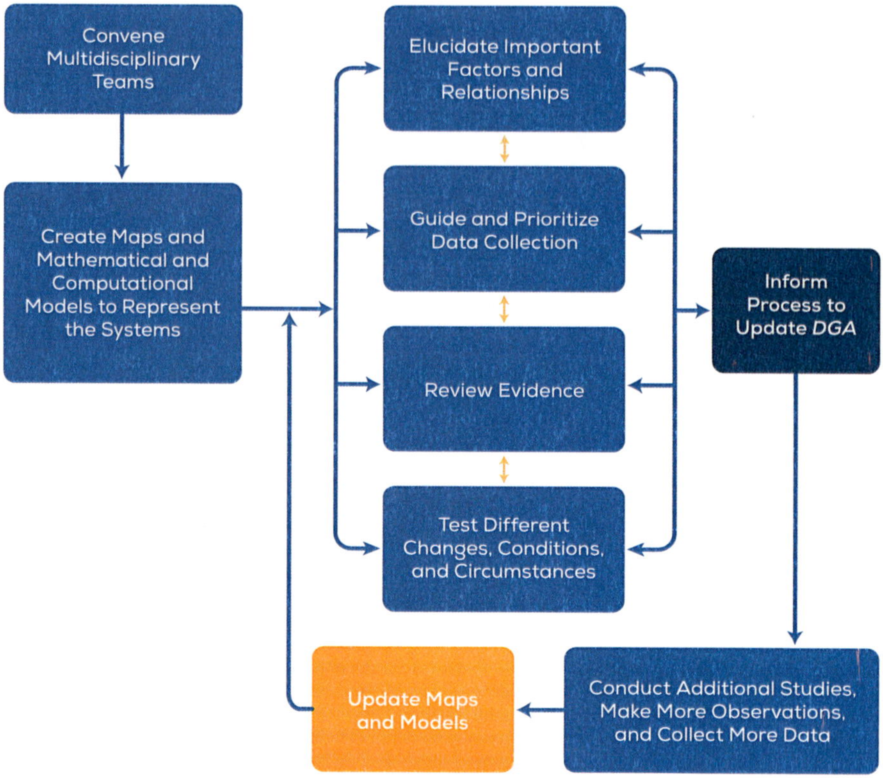

FIGURE 4-1 Iterative process on how a systems approach could be implemented. NOTE: The orange box indicates the cyclical and iterative nature of the systems approach; the dark blue box feeds into the process to update the *DGA*.

DGA involves an organized, iterative process in which an initial systems map is generated, which in turn serves as a blueprint for the systems models. It then guides data collection and study design and implementation, generating more data to further augment and refine the systems maps and models. As Figure 4-1 demonstrates, because the systems involved are complex, fully comprehending these systems will take time over multiple cycles of the *DGA*. An initial representation or model of a system will help guide subsequent scientific exploration and data collection, which in turn can further develop the model.

It may require a few years for systems approaches to be optimally incorporated into the *DGA* process. Although full acceptance, understanding, and integration of systems science will require a sustained, long-term effort, some steps can be taken immediately. Relevant data need to be assembled and catalogued, and modelers with appropriate experience and expertise assembled. Initial systems maps and models will also need to be identified, assembled, or developed. A systems map needs to be created that represents how diet affects health and disease across the variability seen throughout the American population. The systems map will drive the development of the systems models and can then help guide and prioritize data collection. The models will allow for different scenarios to be run (e.g., varying nutritional intakes) to determine what the effects would be. An important, ongoing concurrent process is continuing validation of the models. Typically, validation activities fall into three general types: (1) face validity, (2) criterion validity, and (3) convergence/divergence validity.[9] Sensitivity analyses (systematically varying the values of different parameters) also need to be conducted to help understand the effect of assumptions, uncertainty, and variability in input parameters and the robustness of any results and conclusions.

One hypothetical example of how systems science could be used in nutrition is the relationship between saturated fat and coronary artery disease. Research has suggested that excessive saturated fat intake can lead to lipid deposition within blood vessel walls, initiating a cascade of inflammatory and immune reactions resulting in coronary artery disease. However, there are multiple intermediate steps and potential modifying factors. For example, once ingested, the dietary fat is absorbed through the gastrointestinal tract to varying degrees, which may be affected by local mechanisms and genetic factors. Once in the blood stream, the fat may be further metabolized by the liver in ways that can vary depending on the individual's metabolism, liver function, and genetic predisposition. Further pathways affect how the fat may be transported to the coronary arteries and ultimately deposited. There are also different ways in which blockage of coronary arteries may result in cardiac events. These pathways also do not account for all of the factors and mechanisms outside the body that can modify the way dietary fat affects heart disease (see Box 4-5). Therefore, to fully understand the relationship between fat and coronary artery disease, these pathways need to be outlined in a systems map. Then, mathematical equations need to be developed to represent the dynamics of each of these pathways, including the factors that affect them. Once the initial model is in place, the levels of dietary fat intake can be varied to determine effects throughout the pathways and the result on cardiac outcomes. The process of constructing the systems map and model, as well as running the model, can also help identify knowledge

---

[9] Face validity involves showing a model to different experts to determine whether the model represents what it is intended to represent. Criterion validation refers to how well a model can recreate retrospective, concurrent, or prospective data. Convergence/divergence validation compares a model with other modes (e.g., other models, calculations).

and data gaps. Sensitivity analyses can show the effect of each knowledge gap and thus help prioritize future data collection and studies.

This National Academies committee recognizes that the integration of systems science into the field of nutrition is still early, but it believes more aggressive efforts to deploy and evaluate this science should begin now. While arguments have been made that the integration of systems science needs to wait until more data are available and more research has been conducted, the act of beginning to develop systems maps and models can help identify the types of data that need to be collected and the value of collecting such data. These efforts can begin, even with imperfect data.

Recommendation 7. The secretaries of USDA and HHS should commission research and evaluate strategies to develop and implement systems approaches into the *DGA*. The selected strategies should then begin to be used to integrate systems mapping and modeling into the *DGA* process.

This National Academies committee envisions the nutrition systems mapping and modeling endeavor to be an ongoing process, as described above, either built into an agency or outsourced to an organization with a proven track record in systems approaches. Recognizing that the development and implementation of systems approaches will be gradual, iterative, and occur over a number of years, the foundation for the process will ideally begin with the 2020–2025 *DGA* cycle. To initiate the process, the secretaries of USDA and HHS ought to consider convening a group of experts to develop a strategy for the implementation of systems approaches and systems mapping and modeling in the *DGA*. This National Academies committee envisions a workshop, which includes relevant federal and nonfederal expertise, to discuss the options for integrating systems approaches into the *DGA* and result in strategic short- and long-term plans.

CONCLUSION

The *DGA* are based on the DGAC's conclusions, drawn from the integration of multiple types of analyses. Ensuring that the appropriate conclusions are reached requires that the most current and highest-quality data are used, and that appropriate, validated, and standardized methods are implemented.

Current methods need to be strengthened to better support the development of credible and trustworthy *DGA*. Strengthening the NEL process for conducting systematic reviews will require a multipronged approach. First, clearly delineating the roles of the DGSAC and the NEL staff, as well as incorporating formal peer review, would ensure that appropriate methods are used and would minimize the risk of bias in conducting systematic reviews. Second, enhancing the quality of NEL systematic reviews would necessitate alignment with current best practices. For example, ongoing collaboration with other organizations and training of NEL staff, combined with the technological infrastructure to support new systematic review methods, will need to be supported. The usefulness of food pattern modeling analyses can also be enhanced by accounting for complexity and variability in diets. Similarly, descriptive data analyses that provide valuable information to evaluate diet and health outcomes at the individual and population levels can be improved with the use of methods to standardize and improve data quality. In addition, standardizing approaches across *DGA* cycles, in particular approaches to designating nutrients of concern, would allow for comparisons to be made over time.

Advancing the science underlying the *DGA* requires that new methods be adopted as they become available. The relationship between diet and health is complex and exists within larger and more complex systems. As such, efforts to integrate systems approaches and methods (such as mapping and modeling) into the framework for evidence review would result in a better understanding of the mechanisms involving diet and particular health outcomes.

REFERENCES

AHRQ (Agency for Healthcare Research and Quality). 2014. *Methods guide for effectiveness and comparative effectiveness reviews*. AHRQ Publication No. 10(14)-EHC063-EF. Rockville, MD: Agency for Healthcare Research and Quality. http://www.effectivehealthcare.ahrq.gov (accessed May 31, 2017).

AMSTAR (A Measurement Tool to Assess Systematic Reviews). 2015. *What is AMSTAR?* https://amstar.ca/About_Amstar.php (accessed August 14, 2017).

Balshem, H., M. Helfand, H. J. Schünemann, A. D. Oxman, R. Kunz, J. Brožek, G. E. Vist, Y. Falck-Ytter, J. Meerpohl, S. Norris, and G. H. Guyatt. 2011. GRADE guidelines: 3. Rating the quality of evidence. *Journal of Clinical Epidemiology* 64(4):401-406.

Clarke, M., and P. R. Williamson. 2016. Core outcome sets and systematic reviews. *Systematic Reviews* 5(1):11.

COMET Initiative. 2017. *Core outcome measures in effectiveness trials initiative.* http://www.comet-initiative.org (accessed June 23, 2017).

Dhurandhar, N. V., D. Schoeller, A. W. Brown, S. B. Heymsfield, D. Thomas, T. I. Sorensen, J. R. Speakman, M. Jeansonne, and D. B. Allison. 2015. Energy balance measurement: When something is not better than nothing. *International Journal of Obesity (London)* 39(7):1109-1113.

El-Sayed, A. M., and S. Galea. 2017. *Systems science and population health*: Oxford Scholarship Online. https://global.oup.com/academic/product/systems-science-and-population-health-9780190492397?cc=us&lang=en& (accessed August 13, 2017).

Guyatt, G. H., A. D. Oxman, R. Kunz, D. Atkins, J. Brožek, G. Vist, P. Alderson, P. Glasziou, Y. Falck-Ytter, and H. J. Schünemann. 2011. GRADE guidelines: 2. Framing the question and deciding on important outcomes. *Journal of Clinical Epidemiology* 64(4):395-400.

Heimowitz, C. 2016 (unpublished). *Comments presented at USDA* Dietary Guidelines for Americans *listening sessions: Atkins Nutritionals*. Washington, DC, February 19, 2016.

Higgins, J., and S. Green, editors. 2011. *Cochrane handbook for systematic reviews of interventions, version 5.1.0,* The Cochrane Collaboration. http://handbook-5-1.cochrane.org (accessed August 3, 2017).

Homer, J., B. Milstein, K. Wile, P. Pratibhu, R. Farris, and D. Orenstein. 2008. Modeling the local dynamics of cardiovascular health: Risk factors, context, and capacity. *Preventing Chronic Disease* 5(2):A63-A69.

IOM (Institute of Medicine). 2011. *Finding what works in health care: Standards for systematic reviews*. Washington, DC: The National Academies Press.

Krebs-Smith, S. M., P. M. Guenther, A. F. Subar, S. I. Kirkpatrick, and K. W. Dodd. 2010. Americans do not meet federal dietary recommendations. *Journal of Nutrition* 140(10):1832-1838.

Lachat, C., D. Hawwash, M. C. Ocké, C. Berg, E. Forsum, A. Hörnell, C. Larsson, E. Sonestedt, E. Wirfält, A. Åkesson, P. Kolsteren, G. Byrnes, W. De Keyzer, J. Van Camp, J. E. Cade, N. Slimani, M. Cevallos, M. Egger, and I. Huybrechts. 2016. Strengthening the reporting of observational studies in epidemiology—nutritional epidemiology (STROBE-nut): An extension of the STROBE statement. *PLOS Medicine* 13(6):e1002036.

Lee, B. Y., A. Adam, E. Zenkov, D. Hertenstein, M. C. Ferguson, P. I. Wang, M. S. Wong, P. Wedlock, S. Nyathi, J. Gittelsohn, S. Falah-Fini, S. M. Bartsch, L. J. Cheskin, and S. T. Brown. 2017a. Modeling the economic and health impact of increasing children's physical activity in the United States. *Health Affairs* 36(5):902-908.

Lee, B. Y., S. M. Bartsch, Y. Mui, L. A. Haidari, M. L. Spiker, and J. Gittelsohn. 2017b. A systems approach to obesity. *Nutrition Reviews* 75(Suppl 1):94-106.

Miller, P. E., J. Reedy, S. I. Kirkpatrick, and S. M. Krebs-Smith. 2015. The United States food supply is not consistent with dietary guidance: Evidence from an evaluation using the Healthy Eating Index-2010. *Journal of the Academy of Nutrition and Dietetics* 115(1):95-100.

Mozzaffarian, D. 2016 (unpublished). *Comments presented at USDA* Dietary Guidelines for Americans *listening sessions*. Washington, DC, February 19, 2016.

NCI (National Cancer Institute). 2015. *Usual dietary intakes: Food intakes of U.S. population, 2007–2010*. Epidemiology and Genomics Research Program, National Cancer Institute. https://epi.grants.cancer.gov/diet/usualintakes/pop/2007-10 (accessed May 20, 2017).

NCI. 2017. *Dietary assessment primer*. https://dietassessmentprimer.cancer.gov (accessed June 9, 2017).

Schünemann, H., J. Brožek, G. Guyatt, and A. Oxman, editors. 2013. *Handbook for grading the quality of evidence and the strength of recommendations using the GRADE approach*. The GRADE Working Group. http://gdt.guidelinedevelopment.org/app/handbook/handbook.html#h.33qgws879zw (accessed August 3, 2017).

Shea, B., and D. Henry. 2016. Development of AMSTAR 2. In: Challenges to evidence-based health care and Cochrane. *Abstracts of the 24th Cochrane Colloquium, 23-27 October, 2016, Seoul, South Korea*. Hoboken, NJ: John Wiley & Sons.

Smith, V., D. Devane, C. M. Begley, and M. Clarke. 2011. Methodology in conducting a systematic review of systematic reviews of healthcare interventions. *BMC Medical Research Methodology* 11(1):15.

Sterman, J. D. 2006. Learning from evidence in a complex world. *American Journal of Public Health* 96(3):505-514.

Subar, A. F., L. S. Freedman, J. A. Tooze, S. I. Kirkpatrick, C. Boushey, M. L. Neuhouser, F. E. Thompson, N. Potischman, P. M. Guenther, V. Tarasuk, J. Reedy, and S. M. Krebs-Smith. 2015. Addressing current criticism regarding the value of self-report dietary data. *Journal of Nutrition* 145(12):2639-2645.

Trumbo, P. 2017 (unpublished). *Comments to the committee to review the process to update the* Dietary Guidelines for Americans. Washington, DC, January 29, 2017.

USDA (U.S. Department of Agriculture)/HHS (U.S. Department of Health and Human Services). 2016 (unpublished). Dietary Guidelines for Americans: *Process brief, sections 4–5*. Prepared for the Committee to Review the Process to Update the *Dietary Guidelines for Americans*.

Whiting, P., J. Savovi , J. P. T. Higgins, D. M. Caldwell, B. C. Reeves, B. Shea, P. Davies, J. Kleijnen, and R. Churchill. 2016. ROBIS: A new tool to assess risk of bias in systematic reviews was developed. *Journal of Clinical Epidemiology* 69:225-234.

Whitlock, E. P., J. S. Lin, R. Chou, P. Shekelle, and K. A. Robinson. 2008. Using existing systematic reviews in complex systematic reviews. *Annals of Internal Medicine* 148(10):776-782.

Willett, W. 2016 (unpublished). *Comments presented at USDA* Dietary Guidelines for Americans *listening sessions*. Washington, DC, February 19, 2016.

Part II

Part II of this report describes the process to update the *Dietary Guidelines for Americans* (*DGA*). The first edition was produced in 1980 and has evolved with each 5-year cycle. The 2005, 2010, and 2015 editions are the most comparable in terms of method. Part I of this report emphasized the importance of considering what needs to be done in the future to improve the *DGA*. Part II presents the basis for those recommendations and describes the current process. It also assesses the process and presents key findings. Part II includes three chapters.

Chapter 5 explains the current process for developing the *DGA*, with an in-depth review of the process for creating the *2015–2020 DGA*. An evaluation of the process is also provided in this chapter and serves as the foundation for Chapter 3, "Process Redesign."

Chapter 6 describes and evaluates the process for assessing the various types of analyses used to support the *2015–2020 DGA*. As the base of the recommendations made in Chapter 4, "Strengthening Analyses and Advancing Methods Used," this chapter also serves as the foundation for answering the Statement of Task questions "How the Nutrition Evidence Library is compiled and utilized, including whether NEL reviews and other systematic reviews and data analysis are conducted according to rigorous and objective scientific standards?" and "How systematic reviews are conducted on long-standing *DGA* recommendations, including whether scientific studies are included from scientists with a range of viewpoints?"

Chapter 7 describes how the 2005, 2010, and 2015 editions of the *DGA* approached preventing chronic disease and ensuring nutritional sufficiency for all Americans. This chapter builds the basis for this National Academies of Sciences, Engineering, and Medicine committee's response to the Statement of Task question "How the *DGA* can better prevent chronic disease, ensure nutritional sufficiency for all Americans, and accommodate a range of individual factors, including age, gender, and metabolic health?"

5

Current Process for Developing the *Dietary Guidelines for Americans*: Key Findings

This chapter discusses the current process for developing the *Dietary Guidelines for Americans* (*DGA*),[1] as well as key findings from an assessment of the processes used to develop the *2005 DGA, 2010 DGA,* and *2015–2020 DGA.*

CURRENT PROCESS

The process to update the *DGA* involves a number of steps, beginning with administrative tasks and culminating in the release and implementation of the new edition of the *DGA* (see Figure 5-1).

Administrative Tasks to Begin the *DGA* Cycle

Typically the first step to establish a given cycle of the *DGA* is the execution of a memorandum of understanding between the U.S. Department of Agriculture (USDA) and the U.S. Department of Health and Human Services (HHS). The memorandum indicates which agency will serve as the administrative lead for that particular *DGA* cycle,[2] states the intent to establish the Dietary Guidelines Advisory Committee (DGAC),

---

[1] Refer to Chapter 1, Box 1-1, for an explanation of how the term *DGA* is used throughout this National Academies report.

[2] Responsibility for administrative lead and operational costs rotates between USDA and HHS. For the *2015–2020 DGA*, HHS was the lead agency, while USDA will be the lead for the *2020–2025 DGA* (USDA/HHS, 2017a).

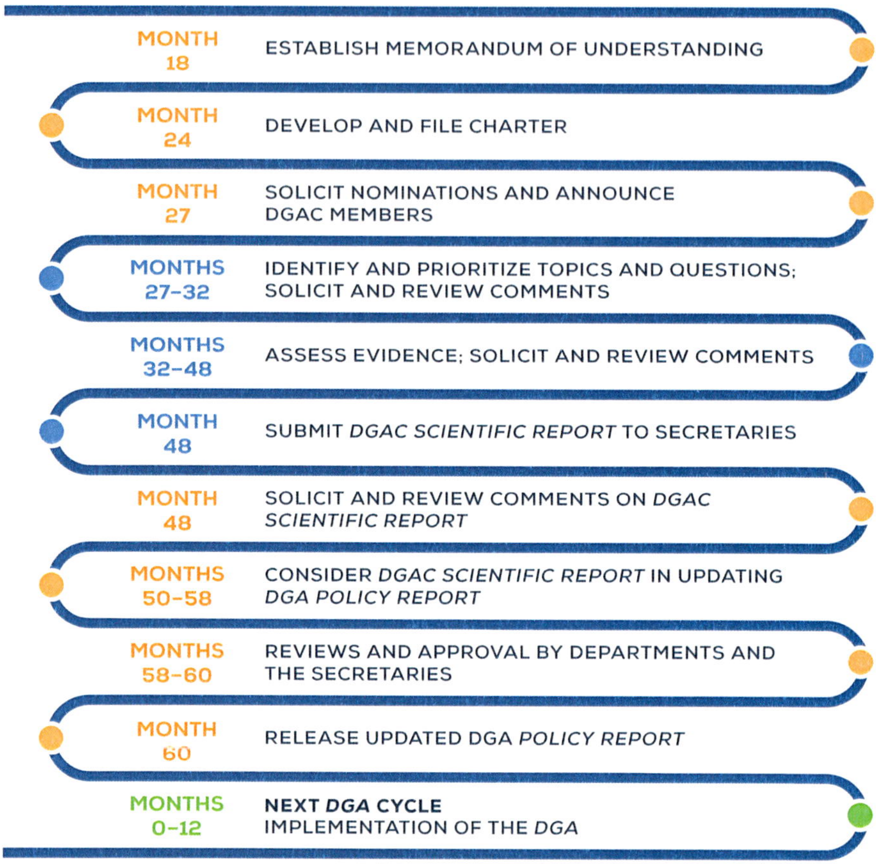
MONTH 18
ESTABLISH MEMORANDUM OF UNDERSTANDING
MONTH 24
DEVELOP AND FILE CHARTER
MONTH 27
SOLICIT NOMINATIONS AND ANNOUNCE DGAC MEMBERS
MONTHS 27–32
IDENTIFY AND PRIORITIZE TOPICS AND QUESTIONS; SOLICIT AND REVIEW COMMENTS
MONTHS 32–48
ASSESS EVIDENCE; SOLICIT AND REVIEW COMMENTS
MONTH 48
SUBMIT DGAC SCIENTIFIC REPORT TO SECRETARIES
MONTH 48
SOLICIT AND REVIEW COMMENTS ON DGAC SCIENTIFIC REPORT
MONTHS 50–58
CONSIDER DGAC SCIENTIFIC REPORT IN UPDATING DGA POLICY REPORT
MONTHS 58–60
REVIEWS AND APPROVAL BY DEPARTMENTS AND THE SECRETARIES
MONTH 60
RELEASE UPDATED DGA POLICY REPORT
MONTHS 0–12
NEXT DGA CYCLE
IMPLEMENTATION OF THE DGA

FIGURE 5-1 Timeline for development of the *Dietary Guidelines for Americans*.
NOTES: Process and timeline based on the *2015–2020 DGA*. "Month" values indicate the approximate number of months after release of the previous edition of the *DGA*, based on an analysis of the *2005*, *2010*, and *2015 DGA* cycles. Orange dots indicate USDA and HHS steps; blue dots indicate DGAC steps; and the green dot indicates steps for government and nutrition and health professionals.

and describes the plan to identify co-executive secretaries. In the past three editions, the memorandum of understanding was executed between 18 and 29 months after the prior *DGA Policy Report* was released.

The next major step is to establish the DGAC. The DGAC is set up as a federal advisory committee, governed by the Federal Advisory Committee Act of 1972 (Public Law 92-463). Before the DGAC can begin its work, a charter must be developed and filed with Congress that states the specific duties and general operational characteristics of the federal advisory committee (GSA, 2011). The charter also lists the categories of expertise sought for on the DGAC. In accordance with the Federal Advisory Committee Act, meetings of federal advisory committees are open to the public unless an exception is granted. Discretionary federal advisory committees generally meet for a period of 2 years after the charter is filed unless (1) otherwise specified, (2) the charter is renewed, or (3) the group completes its work, whichever comes first. The federal advisory committee serves as an independent body for the purpose of providing advice to the government (GSA, 2016).

In establishing the 2015 DGAC, HHS and USDA developed the charge: "Examine the previous edition of the *DGA* and determine topics for which new scientific evidence is likely to be available that may inform revisions to the current guidance or suggest new guidance" (USDA/HHS, 2016a). The DGAC's advice is provided to the secretaries in the form of a report called the *Scientific Report of the Dietary Guidelines Advisory Committee*, referred to in this report as the *DGAC Scientific Report*. The 2015 DGAC comprised 14 individuals selected and appointed by the secretaries of HHS and USDA, representing a broad array of scientific expertise necessary to conduct the work to be performed.

In recent cycles, the charter to establish the DGAC has been filed approximately 2 to 3 years following the release of the prior *DGA Policy Report*. Before the 2010 cycle, the charter was filed prior to the call for DGAC member nominations. The 2010 and 2015 *DGA* cycles followed a slightly different process, where the charter was filed after the call for nominations to give the DGAC more time to conduct its work. For a more detailed discussion of the DGAC selection process, please see this National Academies of Sciences, Engineering, and Medicine (the National Academies) committee's first report (NASEM, 2017). For the 2005, 2010, and 2015 DGACs, members were sworn in and able to begin their work between 6, 4, and 4 months, respectively, into the 2-year timeline, leaving between 19 and 21 months to complete their work. Although five meetings are typically scheduled, additional meetings can be held; the 2010 DGAC met six times, and the 2015 DGAC met seven times.

Identify and Prioritize Topics and Questions

For the 2015 DGAC, USDA and HHS provided some initial guidance for identifying topics, proposing that the DGAC focus on food groups and/or dietary patterns, with an emphasis on food-based recommendations to help promote health and prevent disease. The departments also suggested that specific nutrients only be considered when (1) discussing nutrients of public health concern or (2) advising on how previously established Dietary Reference Intakes (set by the Institute of Medicine) ought to be implemented. Additional guidance stated that topics could be explored if they potentially enhanced how the *DGA Policy Report* was implemented, such as the social, behavioral, and food environmental factors related to diet outcomes such as intake of foods, food groups, and dietary patterns. USDA and HHS also suggested that health outcomes of public health concern ought to be considered by the DGAC, including cardiovascular disease, body weight status, cancer, diabetes, bone health, and prevention of food-borne illness, among others (HHS/USDA, 2013a,b).

To identify topics to consider and address in their scientific reports, DGACs typically divide into smaller groups upon their appointment. These topics are then brought back to the full DGAC for final selection and prioritization. The following paragraphs describe the working structure, which prescribes the preliminary themes for these smaller groups.

The process for developing the DGAC's working structure has changed over time. For the 2005 and 2010 DGACs, USDA and HHS named subcommittees and assigned members to initial subcommittees before the DGAC's first meeting. This initial subcommittee structure was based on a review of the previous *DGA Policy Report* (e.g., guidelines categories from the *2005 DGA* became the initial subcommittees for the 2010 DGAC). Over the course of their deliberations, the DGACs had the opportunity to recast and rename subcommittees or identify additional subcommittees as needed. For example, the 2010 DGAC broadened the scope of the initial subcommittees: the "carbohydrate subcommittee" became the "carbohydrates and protein subcommittee." The 2005 DGAC added subcommittees, such as the macronutrient subcommittee (USDA/HHS, 2016b). The subcommittees for the 2005 and 2010 DGACs had multiple roles, spanning from identifying topics and developing questions to be answered by evidence assessments, to creating plans for reviewing the evidence and drafting conclusions and recommendations for consideration by the full DGAC (USDA/HHS, 2016b).

HHS and USDA recommended that the process be modified for the 2015 cycle by having the DGAC, in collaboration with the DGAC's designated federal officer and co-executive secretaries from HHS and USDA, determine its own working structure with the goals of more efficiently allocating resources and time, and more effectively staffing the DGAC (Millen, 2017; USDA/HHS, 2016b) (see Table 5-1). To accomplish this, the designated federal officer and co-executive secretaries assisted the chair and vice chair of the 2015 DGAC to convene the Science Review Subcommittee, consisting of the chair, vice chair, and two DGAC members who were also part of the 2010 DGAC. This Science Review Subcommittee identified initial themes and assigned the members of the 2015 DGAC

TABLE 5-1 Roles of the Various Working Structures from the 2005, 2010, and 2015 DGACs

DGAC Cycle	Working Structure	Roles
2005 and 2010 DGACs	Subcommittees suggested by USDA and HHS, finalized by DGACs	Identify and prioritize topics; develop questions to be answered by evidence assessments; create plans for reviewing the evidence; draft conclusions and recommendations
2015 DGAC	Three initial work groups	Identify and consider topics; develop questions and topic briefs
	Five subcommittees and additional working and writing groups	Create plans for reviewing the evidence; draft conclusions and recommendations

NOTES: DGAC = Dietary Guidelines Advisory Committee; HHS = U.S. Department of Health and Human Services; USDA = U.S. Department of Agriculture.

to one of three initial work groups: (1) environmental determinants of food, diet, and health; (2) dietary patterns and quality and optimizations through lifestyle behavior change; and (3) foods, beverages, and nutrients and their effect on health outcomes (HHS/USDA, 2015b). The task for each work group was to (1) consider topics of public health concern, informed by the *2010 DGA Policy Report* and *2010 DGAC Scientific Report*, and (2) develop a set of questions based on the importance and likelihood of informing the next edition of the *DGA* (Millen, 2017). In an iterative process, the Science Review Subcommittee edited the work groups' questions, and requested that the three work groups develop topic briefs for each area to help prioritize the many topics. Topics were prioritized through discussion and voted on by all the 2015 DGAC members. These efforts culminated in tiers of topics for consideration that were presented to the full DGAC during public meetings, which also provided the public with an opportunity to comment. Generally, topics and questions assigned the highest priority are then taken up in the next step: evidence assessment (Millen, 2017).

During the 2015 DGAC, the Science Review Subcommittee disbanded the work groups after questions were finalized. The Science Review Subcommittee, in consultation with the designated federal officer and co-executive secretaries, reassigned the 2015 DGAC members to five subcommittees to assess the evidence in regard to specific questions. Subcommittees for the 2015 DGAC included (1) food and nutrient intakes and health: current status and trends; (2) dietary patterns, foods and nutrients, and health outcomes; (3) diet and physical activity behavior change; (4) food and physical activity environments; and (5) food sustainability and safety.

HHS and USDA provided a draft of the topic selection criteria for the 2015 DGAC to consider, which included

1. Target populations;
2. Potential effect on food and nutrition-related outcomes of public health concern, such as health outcomes and diet-related behaviors; and
3. Likelihood of informing recommendations, whether it be to suggest new guidance, inform a revision to current guidance, or address urgent public health concerns (HHS/USDA, 2013a).

These criteria, in addition to a description and rationale for each proposed topic, were included in each topic brief.

Next, the 2015 DGAC considered a number of factors to prioritize among the identified topics. In the committee's first public meeting, HHS and USDA suggested seven criteria for prioritization for the 2015 DGAC:

1. A review of the current evidence on the topic may inform the development of new dietary guidance for Americans ages 2 years and older.
2. A review of the current evidence on the topic may result in a change or elaboration in existing recommendations.
3. The topic represents important uncertainty or a knowledge gap for decision makers.
4. The topic addresses a dilemma in public health nutrition.
5. The topic represents an area where there is a degree of urgency for guidance (e.g., significant area of public health concern, emerging area for public health action).
6. The topic addresses a common practice in public health nutrition for which there is no government guidance.
7. The topic has the potential to inform the development of dietary guidance that is public health oriented (i.e., the promotion of health and the prevention of disease at the population/community level) and not the development of clinical guidelines to use for the treatment and care of individuals with specific diseases and conditions (USDA/HHS, 2017a).

Members of the public were invited to comment throughout the DGAC process through the public comments database. In this way, input on the topics and questions presented during public meetings could be gathered.

The identification, final selection, and prioritization of topics and questions took approximately 5 months for the 2015 DGAC to complete.

Assess Evidence

This section focuses on the general use of the aforementioned subcommittees to assess the evidence. DGACs typically complete their work of evaluating scientific evidence through the use of subcommittees, thereby allowing a number of issues to be discussed at the same time. DGAC members all serve on multiple subcommittees. The 2015 DGAC identified and invited consultants to partake in subcommittee deliberations. These consultants were not members of the DGAC and did not participate in discussions or decisions made by the full DGAC.[3] Two subcommittees of the 2015 DGAC supplemented their own expertise by inviting a total of three consultants to inform their deliberations.

In general, subcommittees conduct their work through conference calls and webinars. For the 2015 DGAC, each subcommittee met on average approximately 35 times. During most subcommittee meetings, members could communicate directly with federal staff who supported the data gathering and analysis efforts of the 2015 DGAC; additional work between the subcommittee and federal staff members, including the Nutrition Evidence Library (NEL), occurred through email.[4] While the subcommittees received support from federal staff and the public in their collection of evidence, the subcommittees independently evaluated the evidence (USDA/HHS, 2017b).

The subcommittees produce assessments of the evidence and drafts of conclusions for consideration by the full DGAC (USDA/HHS, 2016b). Members of the DGAC then work together to finalize conclusions and develop the final report. Additional subgroups of the 2015 DGAC were formed to further advance the DGAC's efforts, such as working on cross-cutting issues. The scope of the subcommittees is subject to change with each cycle. As discussed in the previous section, DGAC subcommittees prior to 2015 were tasked with both developing topics and evaluating the scientific evidence. In contrast, the 2015 DGAC subcommittees focused on examining the evidence, because the topics were identified by the work groups.

The subcommittees' work has also changed as the types of evidence it considers has evolved. The 2010 and 2015 DGACs considered four types of

---

3 While consultants received training and were cleared through the federal process like the DGAC members, they were not members of the full committee and could not vote on decisions made by the DGAC (USDA/HHS, 2016b).

4 Multiple types of federal support staff were involved with the 2015 DGAC. In addition to the co-executive secretaries who represented USDA and HHS throughout the 2015 DGAC process, the Dietary Guidelines Management Team provided administrative support to the DGAC and its subcommittees, the NEL staff helped the DGAC conduct systematic reviews according to NEL systematic review methods, and the Data Analysis Team presented analyses and summaries of data from USDA and HHS as requested by the DGAC.

evidence: (1) original systematic reviews with support from USDA's NEL; (2) existing systematic reviews, meta-analyses, and reports; (3) descriptive data analyses (e.g., intakes of foods and nutrients); and (4) food pattern modeling analyses. The types of evidence have grown with changes in nutrition science. For example, food pattern modeling was first formally introduced for inclusion during the 2005 DGAC, and the NEL was first employed by the 2010 DGAC (USDA/HHS, 2016a). Plans for evaluating the evidence are decided early on by the subcommittees based on the question being asked, some of which require a combination of methods to address. More information about the methods and standards used to assess the evidence can be found in Chapter 6.

Other sources of information that the DGAC considers include expert speakers and public comments. DGACs typically invite expert speakers to their second and/or third meetings. Speakers are also invited by subcommittees to discuss a particular topic during subcommittee meetings; those speakers are announced during the public session of the full DGAC. Public comments are also solicited over the course of the DGAC's work through various channels. Spoken comments can also be made directly to the DGAC, typically during its second meeting; in the past, upward of 53 comments have been made in person. Comments can also be submitted through an online public comments application at any time, where individuals are able to select a topic area under which they feel their comments belong. The 2015 DGAC also issued a call for public comments to ask for submission of literature and evidence related to specific topics, which were to be received early in the DGAC process. Federal staff summarize comments submitted for the DGAC's consideration, typically by topic area. All public comments are also available for general viewing through the online comments database. In total, the 2015 DGAC received 918 comments from the public before the release of its report (USDA/HHS, 2016b).

Submit *DGAC Scientific Report*

The DGAC prepares its findings and conclusions in the form of the *DGAC Scientific Report*. The scientific report is submitted to the secretaries of HHS and USDA and publicly released by the departments. The DGAC creates the report, which has historically been a consensus-based document, with the secretaries of USDA and HHS as the target audience for its advice. The *DGAC Scientific Report* is written by the DGAC itself, with support from a science writer and federal staff. If consensus is not reached, it is up to each DGAC to determine the processes for addressing the differences.

The *DGAC Scientific Report* generally includes an executive summary and a methods section, and the remaining science-based chapters generally describe the evidence assessments. Structurally, the science-based chapters reflect the subcommittee structure. The DGAC chair and co-chair lead the development of the introductory materials and executive summary. Each of the science-based chapters typically includes an introduction, a list of questions examined, a description of methods used, a summary, a list of future research needs, and references. In response to each question addressed, the 2010 and 2015 DGACs included both conclusion statements and implications statements. Conclusion statements directly respond to the questions and summarize the evidence reviewed. Implications statements provide context for the conclusion and generally describe how the DGAC believes its conclusions can be implemented, whether through an action, policy, or other initiative. Research recommendations are also included in the *DGAC Scientific Report*. These generally include emerging issues, research gaps, and limitations of the current body of evidence. In addition to the explanations provided in the scientific report, the DGAC produces online-only appendices to describe its evaluations. Supplementary materials, such as the literature reviewed by the DGAC and detailed descriptions of how food pattern modeling is conducted, are also made available on the departments' websites to promote transparency.

The subcommittees write and review the science-based chapters, which are then edited by a science writer. If a NEL-conducted systematic review is used, NEL staff can review the draft for accuracy of the description. Other DGAC members who are not part of the specific subcommittee authoring the chapter serve as peer reviewers for each chapter. The full draft of the report is typically discussed during the DGAC's final public meeting; only the substantive changes discussed at the meeting and minor editorial changes can be made after the final meeting (USDA/HHS, 2016b). Upon finalizing the scientific report, the DGAC submits it to the secretaries of USDA and HHS; it is then posted on dietaryguidelines.gov. Upon submission of the report, the DGAC disbands.

Solicit and Review Comments on the *DGAC Scientific Report*

No official peer review takes place of the *DGAC Scientific Report*, but after it is submitted, the report is subject to a formal public comment period and a federal interagency review. HHS and USDA also hold a public meeting, announced in the *Federal Register*, about 1 month after the scientific report's release to receive oral comments. Commenters are allowed 3 minutes to address HHS and USDA officials and the co-executive secretaries. Seventy-three individuals provided oral comments in response to the *2015 DGAC Scientific Report* (USDA/HHS, 2016b).

Comments on the *DGAC Scientific Report* are also received through the aforementioned online application and can be accessed by the public at any time. Federal staff process and summarize every comment and filter out any duplicate, blank, or irrelevant comments. In the case of the 2015 DGAC, the public comment period lasted for a total of 75 days during which more than 29,000 public comments were received, 21,000 of which were form letters or petitions (USDA/HHS, 2016b).

A federal interagency review takes place simultaneously with the public comment period, during which *any* federal departments or agencies with nutrition expertise are encouraged to comment, not just those within USDA and HHS. The purpose of the interagency review is to provide feedback and advice to the federal staff who use the *DGAC Scientific Report* as the scientific underpinning of the *DGA Policy Report*. USDA and HHS suggest that review comments submitted by other agencies be based on science, be the consensus view of that agency to facilitate processing of comments, and also provide insight on how the DGAC's recommendations can affect that agency's programmatic policies. Emphasis is placed on comments with scientific justification to ensure that the focus of the *DGA Policy Report* is founded on science, not the number of comments for or against a topic. All comments are considered by USDA and HHS in the next step: the *DGAC Scientific Report* informing the development of the *DGA Policy Report* by USDA and HHS.

Moving from the *DGAC Scientific Report* to the *DGA Policy Report*

Upon publication of the *DGAC Scientific Report*, a joint USDA and HHS writing team is appointed and examines that report as it develops the *DGA Policy Report*. After the report is drafted, it undergoes a series of reviews before release. The amount of time from the release of the *DGAC Scientific Report* to the release of the *DGA Policy Report* has ranged from 5 months, to 8 months, to 11 months for the past three editions respectively.

Dietary Guidelines Writing Team

The *DGA* writing team's role is to accurately translate the "preponderance of scientific evidence"[5]—based on the *DGAC Scientific Report*, public comments, and federal interagency review comments—into language for health professionals and policy makers to advance the scientific basis of federal nutrition programs. The product of the writing team's efforts is a set of guidelines, presented in the new edition of the *DGA Policy Report*.

[5] National Nutrition Monitoring and Related Research Act of 1990, Public Law 101-445, 101st Cong. (October 22, 1990), 7 U.S.C. 5341, 104 Stat. 1042–1044.

To develop the policy report, the writing team reviews the previous edition of the *DGA Policy Report*, the latest *DGAC Scientific Report*, and public and agency comments on the scientific report. Since the 2005 edition, the *DGA Policy Report* has been developed as a technical document with policy makers and health professionals as the primary audience to inform the development of federal food, nutrition, and health policies and programs (USDA/HHS, 2017a). Previous editions were created as consumer-focused brochures (see Table 5-2).

The 2015 writing team consisted of 12 federal employees selected by the co-executive secretaries from the USDA Center for Nutrition Policy and Promotion and the HHS Office of Disease Prevention and Health Promotion, in consultation with agency leadership. A science writer/editor was also a member of the 2015 DGAC writing team. *DGA* writing team members are experts from USDA and HHS selected for both their understanding of the evidence being considered and the DGAC's work, as well as policy applications within the federal government. The writing team is designed to include equal representation from HHS and USDA, and its members have backgrounds in nutrition science, policy, and communications, and are directed not to represent their own personal interests or opinions. The membership of the federal writing team is kept confidential until the new edition is published to minimize any intentional or unintentional attempts to influence the report. During their participation on the *DGA* writing team, members are asked to recuse themselves from participating in activities that could be or could be perceived to be a conflict of interest (USDA/HHS, 2017a).

In conducting its work, the writing team identifies major themes in the *DGAC Scientific Report* and builds on previous editions of the *DGA Policy Report*. The major themes serve as the basis for chapters of the next edition. Central tenets of the writing process include the following:

1. Base the policy report on the totality of scientific evidence, not just on individual studies or opinions (USDA/HHS, 2017a).
2. Address the needs of federal programs and the details needed to allow the program to transform the evidence base into actions focusing on public health (USDA/HHS, 2017a).
3. Consider unintended consequences and how the public might respond and change their behaviors given proposed advice (USDA/HHS, 2017a).
4. Refine language, and use plain language whenever possible to make sure the document is clear and is not misinterpreted. Designers are also consulted in developing the layout and graphic elements to enhance reader comprehension of main concepts (USDA/HHS, 2017a).

TABLE 5-2 Evolution of the *Dietary Guidelines for Americans*

Year	Method for Reviewing the Evidence	Audience	Focus of Guidance	Type and Length of Publication	Number of Guidelines or Key Recommendations
1980	Review of current science by select scientists from USDA and HHS, along with collective expertise of scientific community	Consumers	Healthy Americans (age not specified)	Brochure; 19 pages	7 guidelines
1985	Creation of Dietary Guidelines Advisory Committee (DGAC) outside the federal sector; relied on their collective knowledge of nutrition	Consumers	Healthy Americans (age not specified)	Brochure; 23 pages	7 guidelines
1990	DGAC's collective knowledge of nutrition	Consumers	Healthy Americans, ages 2 years and older	Technical report (48 pages) used as basis for creation of 27-page *DGA* consumer brochure	7 guidelines
1995	DGAC's collective knowledge of nutrition	Consumers	Healthy Americans, ages 2 years and older, to help promote health and prevent disease	Technical report (52 pages) used as basis for creation of 43-page *DGA* consumer brochure	7 guidelines
2000	DGAC's collective knowledge of nutrition	Consumers, policy officials, nutritionists, nutrition educators	Healthy Americans, ages 2 years and older, to help promote health and decrease risk of certain diseases	Technical report (87 pages) used as basis for creation of 40-page *DGA* consumer brochure	10 guidelines (clustered into 3 messages)

2005	DGAC's search and review of the scientific literature, data analyses, food pattern modeling analyses, and other scientific reports	Policy officials, nutritionists, nutrition educators	Americans, ages 2 years and older, to help promote health and decrease risk of major chronic diseases	Technical report (364 pages) and online appendices (124 pages) used as basis for creation of 84-page *DGA* policy document	41 key recommendations (23 for general population, 18 for specific population groups)
2010	DGAC's systematic review of scientific literature using USDA's newly established Nutrition Evidence Library (NEL), data analyses, food pattern modeling analyses, and other scientific reports	Policy officials, nutritionists, nutrition educators	Americans ages 2 years and older, including those at risk of chronic diseases, to help promote health and decrease risk of major chronic diseases	Technical report (453 pages), online appendixes (266 pages), and supplementary information at NEL.gov used as basis for creation of 108-page *DGA* policy document	29 key recommendations (23 for general population, 6 for specific population groups)
2015	DGAC's systematic review of scientific literature using USDA's NEL, data analyses, food pattern modeling analyses, and other scientific reports	Policy officials, nutritionists, nutrition educators	Americans ages 2 years and older, including those at risk of chronic diseases, to help promote health and decrease risk of major chronic diseases	Technical report (567 pages), online appendixes (600 pages), and supplementary information at NEL.gov used as basis for creation of 144-page *DGA* policy document	5 overarching guidelines with 13 supporting key recommendations

NOTES: *DGA* = *Dietary Guidelines for Americans*; HHS = U.S. Department of Health and Human Services; USDA = U.S. Department of Agriculture.
SOURCE: USDA/HHS, 2016a.

The writing team also considers the scope and purview of the *DGA Policy Report*. For example, while the guidelines are to be promoted by each federal agency in carrying out federal food, nutrition, or health programs, how the guidelines are implemented is at the discretion of each agency. As such, conclusions or recommendations suggested by the DGAC proposing how federal programs, policies, or regulations outside the purview of the *DGA* should be changed are not carried forward in the *DGA Policy Report*. To that end, the policy report is developed with the intent of stating not only what Americans should eat to support health, but also why a particular guideline is supported by the science, as well as providing suggestions to help identify how everyone can play a role in making these ideals a reality (USDA/HHS, 2017a). Considerations are also made regarding how a proposed change might affect the food supply, because changes to better align with a proposed recommendation might affect the overall nutritional profile of a food product (Casavale, 2016).

The *DGA Policy Report* includes different types of guidance. Past editions have included guidelines and/or key recommendations. Although there are no official definitions, the term *guidelines* is generally used in *DGA Policy Reports* to highlight overarching guidance, while *key recommendations* further articulate how to meet the guidelines. Key recommendations are generally used to make statements with the strongest scientific evidence or rationale that will not likely result in substantial changes in the face of new evidence. In the 2015–2020 edition, five guidelines (e.g., "limit calories from added sugars and saturated fats and reduce sodium intake") were supported by 13 key recommendations (e.g., "consume less than 10 percent of calories per day from added sugars; consume less than 10 percent of calories per day from saturated fats; consume less than 2,300 milligrams of calories per day of sodium") (USDA/HHS, 2017a). One principle of developing key recommendations is that they ought to be viewed and applied together. For federal agencies, key recommendations can be considered authoritative statements and can therefore be the basis of policies. The guidelines and key recommendations are discussed in the text of the policy report, which also presents the scientific and public health rationale for those statements, as well as any context of technical specifications necessary for explanation or implementation. The chapters of the policy report contain additional context and technical details, while the appendices contain information on both specific topics and technical, often quantitative, details (USDA/HHS, 2017a).

Incorporating Evidence into the DGA

The *DGA Policy Report* is informed by the totality of the science described in the *DGAC Scientific Report*. To that end, if a topic was discussed across several chapters of the scientific report, the writing team considered the implications of all of those statements and how to address them in the new edition. The *DGA Policy Report* is written to accurately depict the strength of evidence, degree of certainty, relevance, and the relationship between nutrition and health. The writing team also takes into account the difference between association and causation, as studies directly determining causes and health outcomes are not always available. Ever since graded conclusions were included in the *DGAC Scientific Report*, the policy report has been able to incorporate specific statements describing the strength of evidence. The body of evidence described in the scientific report underlies the strength of evidence in the key recommendations (see Box 5-1 for definitions of strength of evidence). Statements supporting the key recommendations describe both how much evidence exists and how consistent that body of evidence is.

BOX 5-1
Strength of Evidence Supporting the *DGA* Recommendations as Considered in the *DGA Policy Report*

"*Strong evidence* reflects a large, high-quality, and/or consistent body of evidence. There is a high level of certainty that the evidence is relevant to the population of interest, and additional studies are unlikely to change conclusions derived from this evidence. Topics that are supported by strong evidence often lead to policy recommendations with the greatest emphasis because of the confidence generated by the evidence."

"*Moderate evidence* reflects sufficient evidence to draw conclusions. The level of certainty may be restricted by certain limitations in the evidence, such as the amount of evidence available, inconsistencies in findings, or limitations in methodology or generalizability. Topics that are supported by moderate evidence can support recommendations of varying emphasis, including complementing those with a strong evidence base."

"*Limited evidence* reflects either a small number of studies, studies of weak design or with inconsistent results, and/or limitations on the generalizability of the findings. When only limited evidence is available on a topic, it is insufficient to inform key recommendations. However, policy statements are sometimes useful for topics that have limited supporting evidence, such as when the evidence for those topics reinforces recommendations on related topics that have a stronger evidence base, to clarify that it is not possible to make a recommendation, or to identify an area of emerging research."

SOURCE: HHS/USDA, 2015a.

Neither the guidelines nor the key recommendations are graded. This is in large part because they are based on the underlying body of evidence. The relationship between systematic reviews and key recommendations does not stem from a direct one-to-one ratio. Multiple systematic reviews inform the guidelines, addressing the topic of the guidance from different perspectives. Other sources of evidence for the key recommendations include food pattern modeling and descriptive data analyses; however, the grading rubrics for establishing strength of evidence does not apply to questions answered using these approaches. A focus of the guidance, particularly for the *2015–2020 DGA*, has been on "overall healthy eating patterns supported by evidence evaluating the eating pattern rather than the individual components of patterns; thus, the evidence grade cannot be applied to each individual component within the eating pattern out of the context of the total pattern" (USDA/HHS, 2017a).

Review of the DGA Policy Report

After a draft of the *DGA Policy Report* is compiled by the writing team, the document undergoes three distinct types of review and revision to ensure clarity and technical accuracy: federal expert technical review, external peer review, and departmental clearances.

First, the draft is reviewed by federal scientists with the goal of building consensus across federal agencies with nutrition policies and/or programs. Experts are selected by USDA and HHS officials based on their subject-matter expertise, familiarity with the *DGAC Scientific Report*, and knowledge of federal nutrition programs and policies. The collective expertise of the federal reviewers is intended to cover the array of topics in the draft, as well as the population groups to whom the *DGA* will apply. Names of commenters are removed before the writing team reviews and discusses the scientific merit of proposed edits, although reviewer names and a summary of the comments are made publicly available on the lead department's website. Sections with major substantive changes made in response to reviewer comments can be sent back to reviewers to verify that proposed changes are appropriately made and no new concerns are inadvertently introduced. For the 2015–2020 edition, more than 100 federal subject-matter experts commented on the draft, including staff that supported the DGAC—a process that occurred over 4 months.

The next round of review invites a select panel of external experts to provide a peer review of the draft, as required by the Information Quality Act of 2001 for influential documents not published in peer-reviewed journals. Reviewers provide independent responses to the draft. Steps are taken to ensure reviews are confidential and anonymous. For example, reviewers sign a confidentiality agreement and do not know who the other reviewers are; reviewers' names are also removed when comments are collated before the writing team assesses and discusses the comments. Typically, 4 to 10 individual reviewers familiar with the role of the *DGA Policy Report* are selected from the fields of human nutrition, health promotion, chronic disease prevention, nutrition education, public health, health policy, and systematic review methodology (HHS, 2015; USDA, 2010). Individuals are generally asked to review the draft for clarity and technical accuracy and are directed to refer back to the *DGAC Scientific Report* if any substantive science-based questions arise. Of the seven reviewers for the 2015–2020 edition, three were members of the 2015 DGAC and three others were members of previous DGACs (HHS, 2015).

Once external reviewers identify needed substantive revisions, affected sections of the report can be sent for a second review to federal staff to make sure no new issues were introduced. For the *2015–2020 DGA*, three major revisions were made after the version was externally peer reviewed (HHS, 2016). Names of external peer reviewers and a summary of unattributed comments are available on the lead agency's website after the report is released, per Office of Management and Budget policies (USDA/HHS, 2017a).

The third and final round of review consists of two parts. First, the agency review secures departmental clearances, and then the administration review culminates with approval by the secretaries of USDA and HHS. During the agency review, representatives from each agency within USDA and HHS are asked to indicate the agency's concurrence with the draft; if the agency does not concur, action must be taken before the new edition can be released. If major revisions are made to the draft at this stage, additional reviews and clearances can be required, although one rationale for having the first round of interagency review is to engage relevant agencies before the final clearance process begins. The administration reviews are begun after agency reviews are completed. Generally for USDA, the Office of the USDA Under Secretary of Food, Nutrition, and Consumer Services and the Under Secretary of Research, Education, and Economics formally review the draft, in addition to the Office of the Secretary of Agriculture. HHS reviews typically include the HHS Assistant Secretary for Health and the Office of the Secretary of HHS. Departmental communications and government relations staff from both USDA and HHS are also involved in the final review.

Release

By statute, a *DGA* report must be released every 5 years. The most recent edition remains the definitive nutrition guidance for federal agencies until the next edition is released. The activities around a release differ with each edition, but the release is generally communicated to nutrition and health professionals within and outside of the federal government, the news media, and the DGAC through a variety of channels. Webinars are also held with relevant federal agencies to describe the new edition.

Federal agencies then implement the guidelines and accompanying key recommendations through food, nutrition, health policies and programs, as well as education materials. One major vehicle for disseminating the guidelines is Choose MyPlate, an online resource used to help Americans align their daily food and beverage choices with the *DGA* recommendations.

To ensure consistency across the federal government regarding science-based nutrition information, HHS and USDA maintain a federal interagency working group called the Dietary Guidance Review Committee. This group meets periodically and reviews federally developed materials that contain guidance to the public on diet to ensure their consistency with the *DGA Policy Report*.

Resources

The cost of developing the *DGA* can be separated into the costs related to supporting the DGAC and developing the next edition. Resources for these activities can be further broken down into operating costs and staff support.

The operating costs associated with supporting the 2015 DGAC totaled approximately $905,000. These funds covered travel and per diem, meeting logistics (e.g., meeting space, webcasting), science writer/editor, management of the public comments application, technical support of the public website, and technical support for the NEL. DGAC members served as volunteers and were not paid for their service; however, travel and per diem were provided for the public meetings. The cost of staff support must also be included. In total, 55 federal staff and contractors were listed in the *2015 DGAC Scientific Report*, equating to an estimated 22.2 full-time equivalents (FTEs) over the 2-year period to support the DGAC. The bulk of this support included work by nutritionists, systematic review methodologists, and public health advisors from both USDA and HHS (USDA/HHS, 2017a).

Operating costs related to development of the *2015–2020 DGA Policy Report* largely covered design and production of final products and materials. Activities included making the final product accessible to people with disabilities and producing HTML and PDF versions. Other operating expenses included the use of a science writer/editor and the hosting of a public comment meeting to receive feedback about the *DGAC Scientific Report*. These operating costs totaled $410,000 for the *2015–2020 DGA*

Policy Report. Staff support generally includes the *DGA* writing team and interagency reviewers. Although approximately 10 FTEs drafted the *2015–2020 DGA Policy Report*, the total number of FTEs involved in the development of that report is unknown because of the extent of federal agency reviews and advisors who contributed (USDA/HHS, 2017a).

INCLUSION OF PREGNANT WOMEN AND CHILDREN FROM 0 TO 24 MONTHS OF AGE

Traditionally, the *DGA* have targeted populations over 2 years of age, leaving guidance for pregnant women, infants, and young children to professional societies, such as the American Academy of Pediatrics and the American College of Obstetrics and Gynecology. A change occurred when the Agricultural Act of 2014 mandated that the *2020–2025 DGA Policy Report* include pregnant women, infants, and young children 0–24 months. The inclusion of dietary guidance for pregnancy and infancy is timely because the emerging evidence that supports the developmental origins of disease (Hanson and Gluckman, 2015) has led to a global call to action to reflect the importance of the first 1,000 days of life in order to ensure normal growth and development, to reduce future chronic disease burden, and to promote future health (Shrimpton, 2012; WHO, 2013). For this reason, there is a critical need for optimizing dietary guidance for pregnant women, infants, and children from birth to 2 years. In 2012, HHS and USDA began to evaluate the evidence to support nutrition guidance for infants from birth to 24 months. It is important to understand the process to date to implement this change. The intent of this work was to release a scientific foundation to develop dietary recommendations for infants and young children from birth to 24 months (the B–24 project); this guidance was to have been separate from the *DGA Policy Report* (USDA, 2017b).

The B–24 project was launched in 2012 with plans for four phases. In phase I, the USDA NEL was to be responsible for launching the B–24 project (USDA, 2017a). The objective of the first phase was to identify topics. In phase II of the B–24 project, systematic reviews on the selected topics were to be conducted. In phase III, the systematic reviews were to form the evidence base for the development of unified dietary guidelines for B–24 by early 2018. In turn, the federal agencies could incorporate this guidance into their programs in the final phase. In the original plan, this guidance could be used by the 2020 DGAC for the purpose of including the B–24 population in its scientific report. The B–24 project process was to "be transparent and public input would be collected and considered throughout" (Obbagy et al., 2014). As outlined below, the original plans for the four phases of the project were subsequently revised.

As the first step, the NEL systematic review program convened a workshop in collaboration with the *Eunice Kennedy Shriver* National Institute of Child Health and Human Development, with the goal of informing the process to identify key topics for evaluation. Broad stakeholder input was included through use of a workshop planning group and working groups. After the workshop, the NEL continued liaising with the working groups via teleconference, email, and face-to-face meetings to (1) develop topic nominations, (2) refine systematic review questions, (3) identify crosscutting issues, and (4) create topic briefs that outline key elements of a systematic review framework. This framework was intended as a basis for potential systematic reviews on each topic (USDA, 2017a). The NEL efforts resulted in identification of six topics and questions to undergo trial NEL systematic reviews. The process for topic identification and refinement was published in 2014 (Obbagy et al., 2014; Raiten et al., 2014).

In February 2014, the Agricultural Act of 2014 mandated that the dietary guidance for B–24 be expanded to include pregnant women, along with infants from birth to 24 months (renamed P/B–24) in the *2020–2025 DGA*. USDA and HHS accordingly adjusted their plan, such that topics and questions of public health importance would be explored and some systematic reviews would be conducted for these population subgroups and made publicly available. However, contrary to original plans (Obbagy et al., 2014) specific dietary recommendations *would not* be developed by early 2018 (USDA, 2017b). Rather, an evidence-based document that addresses the six identified topics to undergo systematic review would be produced and be publicly available (USDA/HHS, 2017b). The P/B–24 project is not a formal step of the *2020–2025 DGA* process; the results of the project may be considered by the 2020 DGAC, just as it considers any other systematic review. Calls for public comment have been deferred to the *2020–2025 DGA* process.

The six identified topics for the P/B–24 project to address are

1. What is the relationship between infant milk feeding practices and (1) growth, size, and body composition; (2) food allergies and other atopic allergic diseases; (3) chronic disease; and (4) childhood leukemia?
2. What is the relationship between complementary feeding and (1) micronutrient status; (2) growth, size, and body composition; (3) developmental milestones; (4) food allergies and other atopic allergic disease; and (5) bone health?
3. What is the relationship between exposure to foods and early food acceptance?
4. What is the relationship between maternal diet and infant/toddler food acceptance and dietary intake?

5. What is the relationship between parental and caregiver feeding practices and growth, size, and body composition?
6. What is the relationship between dietary patterns during preconception/pregnancy and (1) risk of gestational diabetes; (2) risk of hypertensive disorders during pregnancy; (3) gestational age at birth; and (4) birth weight standardized for gestational age and sex? (USDA, 2017b).

Responses to these questions are to be made public through the NEL website by early 2018 (USDA/HHS, 2017b).

KEY FINDINGS FROM AN ASSESSMENT OF THE PROCESSES USED TO DEVELOP THE 2005, 2010, AND 2015 EDITIONS OF THE *DGA POLICY REPORTS*

In its first report, this National Academies committee delineated a set of values, which, if taken together, can enhance the integrity of the selection process: enhance transparency, promote diversity of expertise and experience, support a deliberative process, manage biases and conflicts of interest, and adopt state-of-the-art processes and methods (NASEM, 2017). These values are also central to the process of developing the *DGA* and have been adapted for this broader goal (see Chapter 2).

These values were compared to the current process for developing the *DGA*, it is important to note that not all five values are applicable at every step of the process. As a result of this comparison, this National Academies committee found that the integrity of the process could be strengthened. These findings (summarized in Box 5-2) can be categorized into the purpose of the *DGA*; cycle time and component tasks; and transparency and participation. The following sections describe each key finding.

Purpose of the *DGA*

The first key finding is how the overall purpose of the *DGA* is interpreted. There is no clear indication of the considerations used by USDA and HHS to interpret the National Nutrition Monitoring and Related Research Act, or when the purpose of each particular *DGA* edition was developed. As depicted in Table 5-2, USDA and HHS have seemingly taken careful, deliberate steps to infer the purpose of the *DGA* with each cycle, resulting in an evolution of the methods, audience, focus, and type of publication over time.

For example, prior to 2005, the primary audience of the *DGA Policy Report* was consumers, but consumers were no longer an audience after the 2005 edition. Instead, the *DGA Policy Report* was written for policy officials,

BOX 5-2
Findings from This National Academies Committee's Assessment of the Processes to Develop the *DGA Policy Report*

Purpose of the DGA

1. The purposes and audiences of the *DGA* have not been consistently interpreted over time.

Cycle Time and Component Tasks

2. The 2-year term limit imposed by the Federal Advisory Committee Act has put unreasonable time pressure on the DGAC to complete the tasks with which it is charged.

Transparency and Participation

3. The process for identifying categories of expertise to be represented in the DGAC is completed by USDA and HHS without public input or explanations for how the categories were determined.
4. The process for selecting topics and questions to be addressed by the DGAC is not as transparent as it could be and does not support public input.
5. The process for selecting consultants to the DGAC and policies for how they are used are not as transparent as they could be.
6. The process for developing the *DGA* recommendations themselves does not follow standards for a typical guidelines development process and is not a transparent as it could be.
7. The process for considering the *DGAC Scientific Report* to the *DGA Policy Report* is completed internally by USDA and HHS without an accounting of differences between the two reports.
8. The process and approach for addressing population subgroups (e.g., P/B–24) are not as transparent as they could be.

nutritionists, and nutrition educators. Similarly, the focus of the guidance has shifted. In 1995, the focus of the guidelines broadened from just a target population (e.g., healthy Americans ages 2 years and older) to also include effect on health. The focus changed again in 2000, when "decrease risk of certain diseases" was added, which was changed to "decrease risk of major chronic diseases" in subsequent editions (USDA/HHS, 2016a).

While this evolution is understandable in the face of increased chronic disease-related morbidity in the United States and knowledge of the diet–health relationships has advanced, it has led to inconsistencies in the process used to update the *DGA*. For example, this National Academies committee identified more than 10 different statements of purpose in materials related to the *2015–2020 DGA Policy Report*'s purpose and goals (see Box 5-3). Additionally, although the National Nutrition Monitoring and Related Research Act specifies that the guidelines are for the general public, the stated audience of the *DGA Policy Report* after 2000 does not include the general public. This array of purpose statements and audiences could lead to confusion and potentially mistrust in the process to update the *DGA*.

Cycle Time and Component Tasks

Another key finding is the reconsideration of the timeline under which the DGAC has conducted its work. As a federal advisory committee, the DGAC is limited to a 2-year term by the Federal Advisory Committee Act. Unless actions are taken by the departments to extend the DGAC, it is terminated when it produces its report or when its 2 years is completed, whichever comes first. The number of tasks for the DGAC to complete in this fixed time frame has increased over the decades. For example, the scope of the DGAC has expanded (e.g., inclusion of pregnant women and children from birth to 24 months), and there are more types of evidence to assess (e.g., addition of systematic reviews and food pattern modeling), which take time to produce in and of themselves.

The current process has required that the DGAC spends nearly 25 to 30 percent of its available time completing background and preliminary work, such as topic identification and question prioritization. The amount of time between filing the charter and development of systematic review questions for the 2015 DGAC totaled approximately 8 months. As a result, there was less time for the DGAC to focus on assessing the evidence and creating the scientific report.

This time pressure, in the face of the complicated and time-intensive tasks of the DGAC, can be at odds with the goal of producing a final report, potentially reducing the opportunity for a truly deliberative process. While DGACs to date have completed their tasks on time, future DGACs run the risk of not doing so.

Transparency and Participation

A need for greater transparency was identified in six key findings. This National Academies committee recognizes the process for how categories of expertise are selected for the composition of the DGAC as an opportunity to improve the current process. A *Federal Register* notice is published that announces the departments' intent to establish the DGAC

BOX 5-3
Background Statements Related to the Purpose and Audience of the *2015–2020 DGA*

"The main purpose of the *Dietary Guidelines* is to inform the development of federal food, nutrition, and health policies and programs. The primary audiences are policy makers, as well as nutrition and health professionals." (*2015–2020 DGA Policy Report*)

"The scope of the *Dietary Guidelines for Americans* is to address food and nutrition issues that will inform public health action to, number one, promote population health or well-being and/or, number two, to reduce the significant burden of avoidable disease in the U.S. population as a whole or in the special population subgroups." (2015 DGAC meeting 1 transcripts)

"The *Dietary Guidelines for Americans* is an essential resource for health professionals and policy makers as they design and implement food and nutrition programs that feed the American people, such as USDA's National School Lunch Program and School Breakfast Program, which feed more than 30 million children each school day. The *Dietary Guidelines* also provides information that helps Americans make healthy choices for themselves and their families." (Secretaries' statement from *2015–2020 DGA*)

"The *Dietary Guidelines* provides evidence-based food and beverage recommendations for Americans ages 2 and older. These recommendations aim to:

- Promote health
- Prevent chronic disease
- Help people reach and maintain a healthy weight

Public health agencies, health care providers, and educational institutions all rely on Dietary Guidelines recommendations and strategies.

The *Dietary Guidelines* also has a significant impact on nutrition in the United States because it:

- Forms the basis of federal nutrition policy and programs
- Helps guide local, state, and national health promotion and disease prevention initiatives
- Informs various organizations and industries (e.g., products developed and marketed by the food and beverage industry)" (health.gov)

"Report. (1) In general. At least every five years the Secretaries shall publish a report entitled *'Dietary Guidelines for Americans.'* **Each report shall contain nutritional and dietary information and guidelines for the general public, and shall be promoted by each federal agency in carrying out any federal food, nutrition, or health program.**
(2) Basis of guidelines. The information and guidelines contained in each report required under paragraph (1) shall be based on the preponderance of the scientific and medical knowledge which is current at the time the report is prepared." (National Nutrition Monitoring and Related Research Act)

"The *Dietary Guidelines* is an important part of a complex and multifaceted solution to promote health and help to reduce the risk of chronic disease." (Secretaries' statement from *2015–2020 DGA*)

"These analyses will assist professionals and policy makers as they use the *Dietary Guidelines* to help Americans adopt healthier eating patterns and make healthy choices." (Secretaries' statement from *2015–2020 DGA*)

"The *Dietary Guidelines* is designed for professionals to help all individuals ages 2 years and older and their families consume a healthy, nutritionally adequate diet." (Executive summary *2015–2020 DGA*)

"The *DGA* helps the federal government deliver **'consistent, science-based nutrition information and messages to the public.'** The *DGA* provides a platform for consistency in government programs in food and nutrition." (Process brief section 6)

"[The *Dietary Guidelines*] goal is to make recommendations about the components of a healthy and nutritionally adequate diet to help **promote health and prevent chronic disease** for current and future generations." (*2015–2020 DGA*, Introduction)

"[The *Dietary Guidelines*] will assist [health] professionals and policy makers as they use the *DGA*s to help" the general public as well as population subgroups "adopt **healthier eating patterns and make healthy choices."** (Adapted from Secretaries' statement from *2015–2020 DGA*)

"The goal of the *Dietary Guidelines* is for individuals throughout all stages of the life span to have eating patterns that **promote overall health and help prevent chronic disease."** (*2015–2020 DGA,* Introduction)

NOTE: Bolded statements were used by this National Academies committee to help develop the proposed purpose statement introduced in Chapter 2.

and also solicits nominations for the DGAC. Importantly, this notice lists the areas of expertise the departments are considering for DGAC membership, but there is no opportunity for the public to offer comments on the areas of expertise and experience that ought to be included. Selection of DGAC members also occurs prior to the identification of topics for the DGAC to consider. This sequence is questionable in that it is unclear whether the topics selected are indeed the most appropriate topics to be addressed, thus leading to potential uncertainty of the suitability of the DGAC's expertise. The current process is not as transparent as it could be, and does not sufficiently explain how diversity of expertise and experience is achieved. Additionally, as concluded in this National Academies committee's first report, more transparency is needed throughout the selection process and an emphasis ought to be placed on managing both financial and nonfinancial conflicts of interest (NASEM, 2017).

The process by which topics are identified and questions are prioritized can also be questioned. USDA and HHS have encouraged DGACs to explore specific outcomes (e.g., the 2015 DGAC was encouraged to include topics that have the potential to affect food- and nutrition-related health outcomes), without explanation for how or why these outcomes were selected. Currently, only limited public input is gathered, either through the online database or oral statements made during the DGAC's second meeting. No proposed list of topics to be discussed by the DGAC is shared publicly, meaning that the burden is on the public to follow the DGAC's deliberations and public meetings, potentially limiting the ability of the DGAC to engage in a deliberative process with the public about one of the most critical steps in the process. Similar arguments can be made about the process by which the DGAC develops and prioritizes questions to consider. In addition to not being easily accessible for public input, this National Academies committee found it difficult to identify exactly how questions were developed and the criteria against which questions were prioritized, because this work seemed to occur at the workgroup and/or subcommittee level. This lack of public input into the process for selecting topics and questions to address does not take full advantage of expertise within the nutrition community, thus creating the possibility of subject matter imbalance in the composition of the DGAC. This creates the possibility of enhanced bias, both real and perceived.

The identification of consultants is another point where the integrity of the current process can be questioned. Consultants were introduced during a public meeting of the full DGAC, which provided an opportunity for the public to comment off line. The 2015 DGAC was the first DGAC to use consultants. The need for the three consultants was determined by the two subcommittees that used them, and each comment was discussed with the full DGAC. However, consultants were identified by the subcommittees themselves without an opportunity for the public to make comments or suggest other individuals for consideration, nor was an explanation given of the specific purpose and role of the consultants. Although consultants are vetted for financial conflicts of interest and do not vote on decisions made by the DGAC, they have a unique opportunity to influence the deliberations of subcommittees and the DGAC. This National Academies committee concludes that the consultant selection process is not as transparent as it could be, and may lead to the process being unduly influenced by an individual.

This National Academies committee also recognizes the need for transparency in the development of the *DGA* recommendations themselves and the *DGA Policy Report*. The federal writing team is composed of experts with equal representation from USDA and HHS who are selected by the co-executive secretaries and department leadership (USDA/HHS, 2017a). As described previously, writing team members are experts in nutrition science, policy, and communications. However, other considerations regarding how these individuals are selected (e.g., understanding of scientific methods used, political biases, conflicts of interest) is not clear. Five central tenets for writing the *DGA Policy Report* are also outlined, but detailed information on how the tenets are applied and implemented, as well as how the process of developing the updated guidelines based on the *DGAC Scientific Report*, is not readily available. In a typical guideline development process, one group completes the review of evidence, assesses the quality, and develops the subsequent guidelines. Notably, the *DGA Policy Report* differs in that the DGAC is responsible for reviewing and assessing the quality of the evidence while the federal writing team develops the guidelines. The separation in the *DGA* process stems from the Federal Advisory Committee Act and the National Nutrition Monitoring and Related Research Act.[6] The federal writing team ought not be exempted from adhering to explicit and transparent standards for developing clinical practice guidelines. Several groups have established guidance for evaluating and developing clinical practice guidelines that could be consulted as models for the *DGA* process (Brouwers et al., 2010; Guyatt et al., 2008; IOM, 2011; Schünemann et al., 2013, 2014). The process for developing the *DGA* recommendations is not as transparent as it could be, leading to questions about how the evidence was considered and whether the federal writing team was influenced by politics or other factors.

---

[6] The Federal Advisory Committee Act allows federal advisory committees to provide advice to the executive branch; in this case the DGAC can advise USDA and HHS. However, the DGAC would not be allowed to author the guidelines because the National Nutrition Monitoring and Related Research Act requires that the secretaries of USDA and HHS publish the *DGA* every 5 years.

Another limitation of the current process is the lack of transparency regarding how and why decisions were made in the consideration of the *DGAC Scientific Report* when updating the *DGA Policy Report*. The process is internal to USDA and HHS, without an accounting of differences between the two reports or an independent referee to assure the public that reviewers' concerns were appropriately addressed. This opens the process up to criticism that it is subject to undue influences. For example, in the 2015 cycle, while issues regarding sustainability and a proposed sugar tax were determined by the secretaries to be outside the scope, suggestions from the DGAC related to cholesterol were modified. The process for considering each *DGAC Scientific Report* is not as transparent as it should be and does not encourage a deliberative process.

The final key finding of this National Academies committee regarding transparency is that the P/B–24 project process has not been as clear as it could be. The original B–24 project utilized a process to allow for expert and stakeholder input in the identification of key public health outcomes related to nutrition of infants from birth to 24 months. Experts and stakeholders engaged in the process through working groups to help develop and refine questions, and identified research papers that might provide evidence to address those questions. A seemingly similar process was developed for the expanded P/B–24 project. However, specific details of the P/B–24 project were not available to this National Academies committee. For example, the USDA P/B–24 website states that USDA and HHS nutritionists prioritized the aforementioned systematic review questions to be addressed, but there was no mention of input from the broader stakeholder community. Additionally, the NEL is noted to be "collaborating with programmatic and scientific experts in nutrition during pregnancy and early childhood to conduct systematic reviews" (USDA, 2017b), but it is unclear who these experts are or what their roles are in conducting the systematic review. Importantly, it is not immediately evident who will be responsible for grading the evidence from the systematic reviews—NEL staff or these programmatic and scientific experts. Any plans for peer review prior to publication on line are also not shared publicly. Lastly, it is unclear how the goals from the original B–24 project shifted from dietary guidelines to identification of topics and conduct of systematic reviews. The lack of a clear description of how the public has been engaged since completion of work by the B–24 working groups leaves this National Academies committee to conclude that the current P/B–24 project does not take full advantage of all stakeholder expertise within the nutrition community. Articulation of the process for public and stakeholder participation can help reduce uncertainty and strengthen trust and support for the deliberations.

CONCLUSION

The process to update the *DGA* has evolved over time. The approach to evaluating the evidence has been revised to address changes in the health of Americans and the state of nutrition science. New types of science have been introduced, and a new focus of guidance has been addressed; however, the limitations of doing so given the constraints of the process have not been adequately considered. The process needs to be deliberately reviewed and redesigned so that it can adapt to changes in the future. This National Academies committee concludes there are multiple opportunities to improve the process to update the *DGA*, but a comprehensive approach needs to be taken to most effectively achieve the promise of the *DGA*.

REFERENCES

Brouwers, M., M. E. Kho, G. P. Browman, J. S. Burgers, F. Cluzeau, G. Feder, B. Fervers, I. D. Graham, J. Grimshaw, S. Hanna, P. Littlejohns, J. Makarski, and L. Zitzelsberger, for the AGREE Next Steps Consortium. 2010. AGREE II: Advancing guideline development, reporting and evaluation in healthcare. *Canadian Medical Association Journal* 182(18):E839-E842.

Casavale, K. 2016 (unpublished). *Process steps to update and release the* Dietary Guidelines for Americans. Presentation to the Committee to Review the Process to Update the *Dietary Guidelines for Americans*, Washington, DC, October 17, 2016.

GSA (General Services Administration). 2011. *Preparing federal advisory committee charters.* http://www.gsa.gov/portal/mediaId/169411/fileName/Preparing_Federal_Advisory_Committee_Charters_v_2 (accessed March 8, 2017).

GSA. 2016. *When is the Federal Advisory Committee Act applicable?* https://www.gsa.gov/portal/content/100794 (accessed August 9, 2017).

Guyatt, G. H., A. D. Oxman, R. Kunz, Y. Falck-Ytter, G. E. Vist, A. Liberati, and H. J. Schünemann. 2008. Going from evidence to recommendations. *BMJ* 336(7652):1049-1051.

Hanson, M. A., and P. D. Gluckman. 2015. Developmental origins of health and disease—global public health implications. *Best Practice & Research Clinical Obstetrics & Gynaecology* 29(1):24-31.

HHS (U.S. Department of Health and Human Services). 2015. *Office of the assistant secretary of health peer review agenda:* Dietary Guidelines for Americans, 2015. https://aspe.hhs.gov/system/files/pdf/136266/2015%20DGA%20peer%20review%20agenda%20submitted%2012%2016%2015.pdf (accessed February 27, 2017).

HHS. 2016. *Summary of peer-reviewed comments on DGA.* https://aspe.hhs.gov/pdf-document/summary-peer-reviewed-comments-dga (accessed February 27, 2017).

HHS/USDA (U.S. Department of Agriculture). 2013a. *2015 DGAC meeting 1: Topic selection criteria and approaches for examining the evidence.* https://health.gov/dietaryguidelines/2015-BINDER/meeting1/topicSelectionCriteria.aspx (accessed March 12, 2017).

HHS/USDA. 2013b. *2015 Dietary Guidelines Advisory Committee first meeting transcript.* https://health.gov/dietaryguidelines/2015-BINDER/meeting1/docs/Transcript-Day-2.pdf (accessed May 30, 2017).

HHS/USDA. 2015a. Dietary Guidelines for Americans *2015–2020: Eighth edition.* https://health.gov/dietaryguidelines/2015/guidelines (accessed July 18, 2017).

HHS/USDA. 2015b. *Scientific report of the 2015 Dietary Guidelines Advisory Committee.* Washington, DC: USDA, Agricultural Research Service.

IOM (Institute of Medicine). 2011. *Clinical practice guidelines we can trust.* Washington, DC: The National Academies Press.

Millen, B. 2017 (unpublished). *Understanding the committee's methodology for topic formation and reviewing the evidence base.* Presentation to the Committee to Review the Process to Update the *Dietary Guidelines for Americans*, Washington, DC, January 10, 2017.

NASEM (National Academies of Sciences, Engineering, and Medicine). 2017. *Optimizing the process for establishing the* Dietary Guidelines for Americans: *The selection process.* Washington, DC: The National Academies Press.

Obbagy, J. E., D. M. Blum-Kemelor, E. V. Essery, J. M. Lyon, and J. M. Spahn. 2014. USDA Nutrition Evidence Library: Methodology used to identify topics and develop systematic review questions for the birth-to-24-mo population. *American Journal of Clinical Nutrition* 99(3):692S-696S.

Raiten, D. J., R. Raghavan, A. Porter, J. E. Obbagy, and J. M. Spahn. 2014. Executive summary: Evaluating the evidence base to support the inclusion of infants and children from birth to 24 mo of age in the *Dietary Guidelines for Americans*—"the B-24 project." *American Journal of Clinical Nutrition* 99(3):663s-691s.

Schünemann, H., J. Brožek, G. Guyatt, and A. Oxman, editors. 2013. *Handbook for grading the quality of evidence and the strength of recommendations using the GRADE approach.* The GRADE Working Group. http://gdt.guidelinedevelopment.org/app/handbook/handbook.html#h.33qgws879zw (accessed August 3, 2017).

Schünemann, H., W. Wiercioch, I. Etxeandia, M. Falavigna, N. Santesso, R. Mustafa, M. Ventresca, R. Brignardello-Petersen, K.-T. Laisaar, S. Kowalski, T. Baldeh, Y. Zhang, U. Raid, I. Neumann, S. L. Norris, J. Thornton, R. Harbour, S. Treweek, G. Guyatt, P. Alonso-Coello, M. Reinap, J. Brožek, A. Oxman, and E. A. Akl. 2014. Guidelines 2.0: Systematic development of a comprehensive checklist for a successful guideline enterprise. *Canadian Medical Association Journal* 186(3):E123-E142.

Shrimpton, R. 2012. Global policy and programme guidance on maternal nutrition: What exists, the mechanisms for providing it, and how to improve them? *Paediatric and Perinatal Epidemiology* 26:315-325.

USDA. 2010. *Peer review plan for the* 2010 Dietary Guidelines for Americans. https://www.cnpp.usda.gov/sites/default/files/DGPeerReviewPlan.pdf (accessed February 18, 2017).

USDA. 2017a. *Nutrition Evidence Library—birth to 24 months (B-24) topic identification project.* https://www.cnpp.usda.gov/nutrition-evidence-library-birth-24-months-b-24-topic-identification-project (accessed January 8, 2017).

USDA. 2017b. *Pregnancy and birth to 24 months project.* https://www.cnpp.usda.gov/birthto24months (accessed January 8, 2017).

USDA/HHS. 2016a (unpublished). Dietary Guidelines for Americans: *Process brief, sections 1–3.* Prepared for the Committee to Review the Process to Update the *Dietary Guidelines for Americans.*

USDA/HHS. 2016b (unpublished). Dietary Guidelines for Americans: *Process brief, sections 4–5.* Prepared for the Committee to Review the Process to Update the *Dietary Guidelines for Americans.*

USDA/HHS. 2017a (unpublished). Dietary Guidelines for Americans: *Process brief, sections 6–7.* Prepared for the Committee to Review the Process to Update the *Dietary Guidelines for Americans.*

USDA/HHS. 2017b (unpublished). *HMD follow up questions for USDA.* Response to Committee to Review the Process to Update the *Dietary Guidelines for Americans.*

WHO (World Health Organization). 2013. *Essential nutrition actions: Improving maternal, newborn, infant and young child health and nutrition.* Geneva, Switzerland: World Health Organization.

6

Current Approaches to Examining the Evidence: Key Findings

The National Nutrition Monitoring and Related Research Act of 1990 states that the *Dietary Guidelines for Americans* (*DGA*)[1] should provide "nutritional and dietary information and guidelines . . . based on the preponderance of the scientific and medical knowledge which is current at the time the report is prepared."[2] As written in the Statement of Task (see Box 1-3), this committee of the National Academies of Sciences, Engineering, and Medicine (the National Academies) was requested by Congress to review "(2) how the Nutrition Evidence Library (NEL) is compiled and utilized, including whether NEL reviews and other systematic reviews and data analysis are conducted according to rigorous and objective scientific standards; and (3) how systematic reviews are conducted on long-standing *DGA* recommendations, including whether scientific studies are included from scientists with a range of viewpoints."[3] To respond to these requests, this chapter summarizes the approach taken by this National Academies committee to review and evaluate the processes used in examining the evidence that underlies the *DGA* recommendations.

This chapter is divided into sections to reflect the types of analyses traditionally used by the Dietary Guidelines Advisory Committee (DGAC):

---

[1] Refer to Chapter 1, Box 1-1, for an explanation of how the term *DGA* is used throughout this National Academies report.

[2] National Nutrition Monitoring and Related Research Act of 1990, Public Law 101-445, 101st Cong. (October 22, 1990), 7 U.S.C. 5341, 104 Stat. 1042–1044.

[3] Consolidated Appropriations Act, 2016, Public Law 114-113, 114th Cong. (December 18, 2015), 129 Stat. 2280–2281.

(1) original NEL systematic reviews, (2) existing systematic reviews, meta-analyses, and reports, (3) food pattern modeling, and (4) descriptive data analyses. For each type of analysis, this National Academies committee first considered the types of research questions that are relevant for the DGAC; the types of analysis that are appropriate to address these questions; and how the 2015 DGAC's review of evidence was conducted. This chapter then discusses ways in which the process can be strengthened or enhanced to best support the *DGA* in the future. Finally, this National Academies committee considered the necessity for and availability of high-quality data for use in each of the four types of analyses used by the 2015 DGAC.

OVERVIEW OF THE TYPES OF RESEARCH QUESTIONS AND ANALYSES USED BY THE DGAC

This National Academies committee analyzed the questions answered by the 2015 DGAC and categorized the questions in the DGAC's evidence review—inclusive of all evidence types—into three broad groupings: eating patterns, prevalence of disease, and relationships between diet and health (see Table 6-1). In some instances, previous DGACs have used multiple analyses for reviewing the evidence to address a specific question.

To understand the prevalence of disease in the overall population, the DGAC asked a series of descriptive questions. Analyses of U.S. population data were used to estimate the number of Americans living with certain chronic diseases.

Questions related to eating patterns included examination of (1) current patterns of food and nutrient consumption in the United States and (2) how changes in food choices would alter dietary intakes. While these areas are related, three main types of questions were addressed (i.e., descriptive, relational, and predictive questions); the 2015 DGAC used

TABLE 6-1 Types of Research Questions Asked and Examples from the *2015 DGAC Scientific Report*

Categories of Questions	Types of Research Questions Asked and Examples from the *2015 DGAC Scientific Report*	Analyses Conducted by the 2005, 2010, and 2015 DGACs
Eating Patterns		
1a. Examine eating patterns in overall population and population subgroups	Descriptive questions Ex: What are current consumption patterns of nutrients from foods and beverages by the U.S. population?	• Descriptive data analyses based on U.S. population data from NHANES (see Table 6-5)

TABLE 6-1 Continued

Categories of Questions	Types of Research Questions Asked and Examples from the *2015 DGAC Scientific Report*	Analyses Conducted by the 2005, 2010, and 2015 DGACs
1b. Examine projected changes in eating patterns (may be based on potential DGAC conclusions)	Predictive questions Ex: How well do the USDA Food Patterns meet the nutritional needs of children 2 to 5 years of age, and how do the recommended amounts compare to their current intakes? Given the relatively small empty calorie limit for this age group, how much flexibility is possible in food choices?	• Food pattern modeling based on U.S. food and nutrient intake data from NHANES and supplemental sources (see Table 6-5)
Prevalence of Disease		
2. Examine prevalence of disease in overall population and population subgroups	Descriptive questions Ex: What is the current prevalence of overweight/obesity and distribution of body weight, body mass index (BMI), and abdominal obesity in the U.S. population and in specific age, sex, race/ethnicity, and income groups?	• Descriptive data analyses based on U.S. population data from NHANES and supplemental sources (see Table 6-5)
Relationships Between Diet and Health		
3a. Examine relationships between diet and health and disease outcomes of interest (e.g., type of relationship, importance)	Relational questions Ex: What is the relationship between sodium intake and blood pressure in adults?	• Literature review/collection of published literature • Systematic review—de novo or update of existing • Existing consensus reports
3b. What interrelationships exist between different types of nutrient intakes (e.g., the combined effect of sodium and potassium versus individual effects)?	Ex: What effect does the interrelationship of sodium and potassium have on blood pressure and cardiovascular disease outcomes?	• Literature review/collection of published literature • Systematic review—de novo or update of existing • Existing consensus reports

NOTES: This table summarizes approaches the 2005, 2010, and 2015 DGACs have taken in their evidence reviews, including the types of research questions asked. It does not offer all possible types of analyses that could be used to answer these questions. DGAC = Dietary Guidelines Advisory Committee; NHANES = National Health and Nutrition Examination Survey; USDA = U.S. Department of Agriculture.

four general types of analyses to answer the questions. To evaluate current eating patterns, the 2015 DGAC asked descriptive questions about the food and nutrient intakes of Americans. These were answered using analyses of U.S. population data such as the National Health and Nutrition Examination Survey (NHANES). To project the effect of changes in eating patterns, predictive questions were asked to anticipate potential outcomes. These types of questions have been addressed through food pattern modeling, a kind of analysis that predicts the effect of the recommended changes.

Given the DGAC's mandate to "promote health and prevent disease," of particular interest and concern for the 2015 DGAC were relationships between diet and health and disease outcomes (including the nature of the relationships, as well as intermediate outcomes) (HHS/USDA, 2015b). Therefore, many of the questions answered by the 2015 DGAC were relational questions. These questions were answered using original systematic reviews, and/or existing systematic reviews, meta-analyses, and reports in the literature.

Methodological Approaches to Different Types of Questions

Over time, the types of analyses used by DGACs to develop the scientific basis for the *DGA* have evolved. Descriptive data analyses were available for use by the DGAC since the origin of the guidelines, but data on dietary intakes were only formally considered by the DGAC as recently as 2010. Food pattern modeling was available and used to produce recommended intakes of food groups since the 1990 edition. Relationships between diet and health were historically based on ad hoc expert examination of the existing literature. However, as the science of evidence review evolved, more standardized methods of systematic review have been considered and employed in the DGAC's review of the evidence. The NEL was introduced in the 2010 cycle. The 2015 DGAC used the following types of analyses:

- NEL systematic reviews: Comprehensive reviews of the literature that adhere to established principles, as well as updates of existing systematic reviews
- Existing sources of evidence: Evaluations of sources of evidence such as published systematic reviews, meta-analyses, and reports
- Food pattern modeling: A type of sensitivity analysis that incorporates various data inputs, constraints, goals, and assumptions to inform food patterns and resulting nutrient profiles, as well as to answer various questions regarding the effects of modifications to food patterns

- Descriptive data analyses: A type of analysis used to answer descriptive questions about overall population trends and population subgroups

DGACs have also considered invited expert testimonies and public comments.

ASSESSMENT OF SYSTEMATIC REVIEW METHODS

Systematic reviews provide a synthesis of relevant existing research on a particular topic.[4] Systematic reviews are a significant source of evidence for the DGAC. Prior to 2010, DGACs relied on existing reports available in the published literature, or drew conclusions based on their own review of the evidence. The NEL is a program housed in the U.S. Department of Agriculture (USDA) Center for Nutrition Policy and Promotion, and it conducts systematic reviews to inform federal nutrition policy and programs (USDA, 2017). It was developed in part to provide support, as well as a structure and protocol, for the DGAC to conduct original systematic reviews (USDA/HHS, 2016).

The use of systematic reviews has varied across cycles with respect to the use of original and existing systematic reviews, meta-analyses, and reports. The 2005 DGAC answered around 44 percent of questions with an evidence-based literature review (17 out of 32 total questions), and roughly the same percentage with existing publications. With the introduction of the NEL in 2010, the number of systematic reviews used by the DGAC increased. During the 2010 cycle, 76 percent of the questions (44 out of 59 total questions) were answered by an original systematic review, while existing publications were used to answer about 12 questions (20 percent). In the *2015–2020 DGA*, 25 percent of the questions (23 of 91 total questions) were answered by an original systematic review, while existing publications were used to answer 44 percent of the questions (40 of 91 total questions).[5] Notably, systematic review methodology has become increasingly common, and thus more reviews were likely available for use by the DGAC in 2015 than in 2010. Despite some variation across *DGA* cycles, systematic reviews, both previously existing and conducted de novo, have served as a key source of evidence. The devel-

[4] Systematic reviews are designed to answer a specific question(s). The DGAC process for selecting and refining topics precedes the development of systematic review questions and is described in detail in Chapter 5. Systematic review questions are developed according to the criteria outlined below in Step 1 of the NEL process.

[5] These numbers were calculated based on the 2005, 2010, and 2015 DGAC reports. See Appendix C for a complete list of questions answered by the 2015 DGAC.

opment of the NEL has led to centralization and standardization of the systematic review process across the most recent *DGA* cycles.

Questions That Systematic Reviews Are Intended to Address

Systematic reviews provide important insights into the relationships between diet and health. For example, such questions as "What is the relationship between dietary patterns and risk of cancer?" and "What is the relationship between sodium intake and cardiovascular disease outcomes?" were the subject of two systematic reviews in the *2015 DGAC Scientific Report*. This type of question intends to assess the stated relationship between a particular aspect of diet within a defined population, with respect to a particular intervention and defined health outcome, and with consideration for known potential confounders. Using systematic reviews to understand the nature and types of these relationships also means distinguishing between causality and associations, depending on the study types and data available. The quality of the studies available may also limit the ability to make certain inferences, and careful consideration of quality and risk of bias of included studies in systematic reviews is important.

The 2015 DGAC also used systematic reviews to consider the relationships of other factors influencing diet and/or affecting health outcomes of interest. For example, the questions "What is the relationship between neighborhood and community access to food retail settings and weight status?" and "What is the impact of obesity prevention approaches in early care and education programs on the weight status of children ages 2 to 5 years?" consider weight status as a health outcome of interest.

Questions of relationship can also be developed in such a way to assess the effect of a particular dietary factor on a health or disease outcome, including intermediate outcomes. Examples of this type of question include "What effect does the interrelationship of sodium and potassium have on blood pressure and cardiovascular disease outcomes?" from the *2015 DGAC Scientific Report*, and, "What are the effects of dietary stearic acid on LDL cholesterol?" from the *2010 DGAC Scientific Report*.

According to NEL protocol, systematic review questions are developed and prioritized in advance of the decision to use an existing systematic review, meta-analysis, or report, or to conduct a de novo systematic review. The process of identifying, evaluating, and deciding whether or not an existing systematic review should be included or excluded requires a different set of considerations than conducting an original systematic review (see "Assessment of the NEL Process for Using Existing Systematic Reviews, Meta-Analyses, and Reports" beginning on page 167).

The USDA Nutrition Evidence Library and Its Approach to Conducting Original Systematic Reviews for the DGAC

The NEL is staffed by nutrition scientists and research librarians with systematic review expertise; for both the 2010 and 2015 DGACs, NEL staff provided support for all original (de novo) systematic reviews.

The design of the NEL protocol for original systematic reviews is based on published methodologies from the Agency for Healthcare Research and Quality (AHRQ), Cochrane, the Academy of Nutrition and Dietetics, and the Institute of Medicine (IOM) (USDA/HHS, 2016). Standardized methodology and protocols are used for the purpose of promoting transparency, minimizing bias, and ensuring the development of high-quality systematic reviews. For original NEL systematic reviews, the review team is composed of the following:

- A DGAC subcommittee (four to seven members), for the purpose of providing expertise specific to the review topic and knowledge of the field;
- One or more NEL analysts, who assist the DGAC in planning, facilitating, conducting, and documenting the systematic review to ensure alignment with NEL methodology;
- One or more NEL librarians, who manage the development, implementation, refinement, and documentation of the search strategy; and
- NEL abstractors, individuals with advanced degrees in nutrition or a related field, who assist in data extraction and risk of bias assessment.

The size of the systematic review team varies based on the project's needs, but at a minimum, one librarian and one analyst are assigned a lead role.

NEL librarians and analysts are required to be trained in systematic review methodology. New staff members are required to undergo approximately 150 hours of training over the course of several months before independently performing any of the steps in the systematic review process (USDA/HHS, 2016). NEL abstractors receive approximately 10 initial hours of training from the NEL staff and an email orientation to the specific systematic review project, as well as ongoing training as needed throughout the project. Prior to approval for participation, evidence abstractors are required to disclose potential financial, professional, and intellectual conflicts of interest (USDA/HHS, 2016).

The six steps in the NEL original review process are as follows:

1. Topic identification and systematic review question development;
2. Literature search, screening, and selection;

3. Data extraction and risk of bias assessment;
4. Evidence description and synthesis;
5. Conclusion statement development and evidence grading; and
6. Identification of research recommendations.

The DGAC makes all substantive decisions during each step, while NEL staff assists in executing and documenting those decisions and ensuring that the process adheres to established NEL methodology. Table 6-2 provides an overview of each step in the process, specifying the roles of the NEL staff, DGAC, and tools used. Even for the steps in Table 6-2 that specify the NEL as the primary actor, the DGAC still provides oversight and direction, and reviews and approves products.

Step 1: Topic Identification and Systematic Review Question Development

Topics are identified by the DGAC. During the topic identification process, the DGAC determines additional information about the topic, including the target population, public health outcomes of interest, and relevant references as appropriate.

The U.S. Department of Health and Human Services (HHS) and USDA suggest topic selection criteria, based on the scope and purpose of the DGAC. These criteria focus on the role of the *DGA* to inform public health action and policy in promoting population health and reducing the risk of disease (Millen, 2017). Also taken into consideration is the likelihood that the results of including the topic in an evidence review will: "(1) inform decisions about federal public health food and nutrition policies and programs, or (2) represent an area of major public health concern, uncertainty, and/or a knowledge gap that is critical to public health policy" (USDA/HHS, 2016). Both scope and importance are considered in selecting topics.

For each suggested topic, the rationale for review, target population, and public health outcomes of interest are outlined, and the approach for examining the evidence for the topic is recommended by the DGAC. These steps apply to all topics, regardless of the type of analysis used to examine the evidence (i.e., original NEL systematic review; existing high-quality systematic reviews, meta-analyses, and report(s); food pattern modeling; descriptive data analyses).

If requested by the DGAC, the NEL provides support at this initial stage of the evidence assessment by conducting exploratory searches. The goals of exploratory searches are to determine whether sufficient evidence is available to warrant a systematic review, to refine search terms and health outcomes of interest, and to provide information to estimate the

TABLE 6-2 Overview of NEL Systematic Review Steps

NEL Systematic Review Steps	Primary Actor	Tools Used[a]
Step 1		
Identify topics	DGAC	N/A
Develop questions	DGAC	PICO
Prioritize questions	DGAC	N/A
Develop analytic framework	DGAC	PICO, key definitions, potential confounders, related questions
Step 2		
Refine inclusion/exclusion criteria	DGAC	N/A
Develop search strategy	NEL	N/A
Screen and select studies	NEL	N/A
Determine inclusion of existing systematic reviews/meta-analyses/reports[b]	NEL	AMSTAR
Step 3		
Extract data	NEL	N/A
Assess risk of bias	NEL	NEL BAT
Step 4		
Synthesize and evaluate evidence	DGAC	N/A
Draft evidence description and synthesis	NEL	N/A
Step 5		
Draft conclusion statement	DGAC	N/A
Grade body of evidence/conclusion statement	DGAC	NEL Grading Rubric
Step 6		
Identify research recommendations	DGAC	N/A

NOTE: AMSTAR = Assessing the Methodological Quality of Systematic Reviews; BAT = Bias Assessment Tool; DGAC = 2015 Dietary Guidelines Advisory Committee; N/A = not applicable; NEL = Nutrition Evidence Library; PICO = population, interventions/exposures, comparators, and intermediate and/or health or dietary outcomes of interest.

[a] For the purposes of this table, this column notes only specialized tools. NEL protocol specifies the methods used at each of these steps, which are outlined in detail in the text.

[b] If no existing systematic reviews, meta-analyses, or reports are identified in the literature search, this step is omitted.

time and resources needed for a systematic review on a specific topic. It is not to provide details on results or conclusions.

For topics that are selected to be addressed with systematic reviews—either original NEL systematic reviews, or existing high-quality reports when available—questions are developed by the DGAC with assistance from federal staff according to the PICO (population, intervention/exposure, comparator, and outcome of interest) framework. The PICO framework outlines the following elements of interest to be included in the question: target population and subpopulations, the intervention and/or exposure, the main comparator, and selected outcomes. Systematic review questions are reviewed and further refined in an iterative process, integrating input from the DGAC to ensure appropriate focus and specificity. The subsequent development of an analytic framework is intended to ensure that the final systematic review question(s) considered critical elements that may have affected the outcome. In addition to the PICO elements, the analytic framework for each systematic review includes key definitions, potential confounders, and a list of all systematic review questions for a particular topic, if more than one was asked. The analytic framework serves as a visual representation of the overall scope of the project and is available publicly during DGAC meetings, online after DGAC meetings, and once the systematic review is completed and the *DGAC Scientific Report* is released.

Step 2: Literature Search, Screening, and Selection

Search For each systematic review project, the lead NEL librarian, working in collaboration with the DGAC and NEL analyst(s), is responsible for developing a search strategy to identify relevant literature and for documenting the search terms, electronic databases searched, and appropriate search refinements.

First, DGAC subcommittees establish a priori inclusion and exclusion criteria for each systematic review based on a set of standard criteria developed by the NEL for the purposes of promoting consistency across systematic reviews and ensuring relevance to the U.S. population. These criteria can be revised by the DGAC subcommittee members if needed based on the topic of the systematic review to address any unique considerations. For example, questions examining the relationship between community food environments or food access and weight status are limited to only include U.S. populations, but for questions on relationships between dietary patterns and cancer, the population is expanded to include individuals from countries with a high or very high human development index (as defined according to the 2012 Human Development Index) (HHS/USDA, 2015b). To promote objectivity and minimize opportunity for bias, any post hoc revisions to the criteria are discouraged by the NEL protocol, and if changes have to be made, the date and justification for the revision are documented in the search strategy.

The NEL inclusion and exclusion criteria cover study design, risk of bias, language, publication status, and health status of study subjects, along with the rationale for selections (USDA/HHS, 2016). Specifically, the standard criteria for DGAC systematic reviews include studies published in English in peer-reviewed journals in generally healthy populations, including populations with elevated chronic disease risk, or a mix of individuals with and without the disease or health outcome of interest. Studies are excluded if they were conducted in exclusively diseased populations or nongeneralizable subsets of the population, were unpublished or in the grey literature, or were published in languages other than English. Studies are not excluded based on a risk of bias assessment, although this is considered in later grading of the overall quality of the evidence (USDA/HHS, 2016). Study designs that are included and excluded may be dependent on the most appropriate design feasible for addressing a particular topic or question. However, standard NEL protocol states that randomized and nonrandomized controlled trials, prospective and retrospective cohort studies, case-control studies, and pre/post studies with a control are included, while cross-sectional studies, uncontrolled studies, pre/post studies without a control, and narrative reviews are excluded (USDA/HHS, 2016). Existing systematic reviews and meta-analyses are identified in a duplication assessment and may be used at the discretion of DGAC subcommittees to replace or augment an original NEL systematic review.

To test the search strategy and identify any potential errors, the NEL librarian performs a preliminary search in PubMed, using PubMed operators and search terms, and previews the results. The search strategy is then peer reviewed by another NEL librarian for the following elements:

1. "The accuracy of translating the research questions into search concepts and terminology;
2. Proper use of search operators, fields, limiters or filters, and spelling of syntax of search terms/strings;
3. The accuracy of adapting the search strategy for each database;
4. Inclusion of relevant subject headings such as Medical Subject Headings (MeSH) with free-text terms; and
5. Provision of additional relevant search terms and/or original databases" (USDA/HHS, 2016).

The NEL librarian makes any necessary revisions during the peer-review process, shares the search strategy with the DGAC subcommittee for review, and subsequently finalizes the search strategy after all additional revisions noted by the DGAC subcommittee are made. PubMed, Embase, and Cochrane are the standard databases searched, but other topic-specific databases may be searched depending on the research question (USDA/HHS, 2016). All databases searched are listed in the search plan and results. The final search is conducted in the selected electronic databases.

Screening The results of the search are independently screened by two NEL analysts via title, abstract, and full-text review. The goal of screening is to review the search results and determine whether each article meets the inclusion and exclusion criteria. A third analyst or member of the DGAC is available to resolve conflicts between the two analysts.

Selection The resulting list of included and excluded articles is reviewed and approved by the DGAC subcommittee. A manual search of the reference sections of included articles is also performed to ensure all relevant articles are included, and to identify any potential gaps in the search.

Duplication assessment Depending on the topic and literature identified, NEL staff can conduct a duplication assessment to identify any existing high-quality systematic reviews, meta-analyses, or reports that answer the systematic review topic or question of interest. Existing systematic reviews, meta-analyses, and reports may be used to either replace an original systematic review or to supplement a systematic review as an additional source of evidence.

If an existing systematic review, meta-analysis, or report is identified during the search and screening process, the DGAC subcommittee is responsible for determining if and how it should be used, based on the report's relevance to the systematic review question of interest, the quality of the report, the timeliness of the report, and with consideration for reference overlap. The assessment is based on PICO elements, AMSTAR rating, and the date range of the existing systematic review (see "Assessment of the NEL Process for Using Existing Systematic Reviews, Meta-Analyses, and Reports" beginning on page 167 for more information). If multiple existing reports are identified on the same topic and the conclusions are similar, the NEL can combine them in consideration of overall evidence; if conclusions differ, they can be used for background information, but are not deemed an appropriate source of evidence. If no existing high-quality reports are identified, the NEL proceeds with an original systematic review on the identified topic and questions.

Step 3: Data Abstraction and Risk of Bias Assessment

In preparation for the review and summary of the evidence, data relevant to the systematic review question are extracted and risk of bias is assessed for each article included in a systematic review. A standardized evidence extraction form is developed by the NEL analyst and approved by the DGAC subcommittee to ensure all relevant data are collected. These forms are organized generally by study characteristics, participant characteristics, exposure(s)/independent variable(s), outcome(s)/dependent variable(s), limitations/risks of bias, funding, and related articles. Specific instructions are also provided to ensure all relevant information is collected (e.g., for Dietary Assessment Method, example instructions may specify: "enter name and/or type of instrument used and a brief description of tool, if it was validated for the study sample, number of data collection points, and which data points were used for diet assessment") (USDA/HHS, 2016). Data extraction can be done with assistance from NEL abstractors.

After completing the data extraction, risk of bias (internal validity) in individual studies is assessed using the NEL Bias Assessment Tool (BAT). The NEL BAT was developed to assess the risk of bias of individual studies included in NEL systematic reviews, and is based on existing risk of bias tools, including those developed by the Agency for Healthcare Research and Quality and Cochrane, and follows a question/answer format (Higgins and Green, 2011; USDA/HHS, 2016; Viswanathan et al., 2012, 2013; West et al., 2002). The tool is designed to assess four types of bias, including

1. Selection bias, through assessment of inclusion/exclusion criteria, recruitment, allocation of participants, and baseline distribution of confounders;
2. Performance bias, through assessment of adherence to study protocol by the participants and investigators, unplanned concurrent exposures, and blinding of the participants and investigators;
3. Detection bias, through assessment of blinding of the outcome assessors, outcome measures, and statistical methods; and
4. Attrition bias, through assessment of follow-up length and attrition (high/differential).

Each of these assessments is facilitated by a set of targeted questions specific to randomized controlled trials, nonrandomized controlled trials, or observational studies. For example, to assess blinding of participants on randomized or nonrandomized controlled trials, the NEL BAT question is "Were participants blinded to their intervention or exposure status?" Each question can be answered with one of four responses: yes, no, cannot determine, and not applicable. NEL protocol specifies that "yes" or "no" responses should be selected if sufficient information is provided in the study to clearly indicate the answer to the question; if no or insufficient information is available in the study, "cannot determine" should be selected; and "not applicable" should be selected if the question is not applicable to the study. For quality control purposes, the NEL BAT is completed in a dual process where both the evidence abstractor and an NEL analyst independently complete the bias assessment. Any conflicts identified are to be resolved by the abstractor and analyst, with assistance from another NEL staff member, if needed (USDA/HHS, 2016).

The analyst combines the extracted data and limitations identified via the NEL BAT into a spreadsheet referred to as the evidence grid to assist the DGAC subcommittee's review of the evidence (USDA/HHS, 2016).

Step 4: Evidence Description and Synthesis

The DGAC subcommittee reviews the evidence grid and the full-text manuscripts of the articles identified in the search. This review is facilitated by a series of probing questions provided by the NEL analyst, referred to as the evidence portfolio worksheet, which are independently completed by each DGAC subcommittee member. These questions vary in their focus and aim and are intended to aid the DGAC members in comparing and contrasting the studies reviewed, and to assist with subsequent development of a conclusion statement along with a grade of the overall quality of the evidence. Some of the questions are intended to evaluate the characteristics affecting the quality of the study and potential considerations, and include the following:

- "Whether the reported effects of a study are likely to be the true effects of the intervention/exposure,
- Whether the sample size of a study is sufficient to avoid type I and II errors,
- Whether a study is designed to directly examine the link between the intervention/exposure and the outcome(s) of interest in the systematic review question, and
- Whether a study is generalizable to the U.S. population of interest" (USDA/HHS, 2016).

Other questions focus on the specific intervention/exposure and outcome(s) of interest for the systematic review. Study limitations, consistency of results, methodological differences resulting in disagreement in outcomes, significance of results, and reliability across multiple independent research groups are also noted.

The NEL analyst compiles information from the DGAC subcommittee's review of the evidence portfolio to facilitate drafting of the evidence description and synthesis by a DGAC member(s) or the analyst, which includes descriptive information about the review and a summary of findings. The draft synthesis of evidence is reviewed by the DGAC subcommittee; a minimum of three subcommittee members are required to provide feedback before the synthesis can move forward (USDA/HHS, 2016). The synthesis of evidence generally compares and contrasts the interventions/exposures and outcome(s) of interest, methodology, and results. Also included in the final evidence synthesis is a discussion of the themes of the systematic review question, an overview table providing a summary of the results and key study characteristics, an assessment of the body of evidence according to the aspects outlined in the NEL grading rubric, and the resulting research recommendations and rationale.

Step 5: Conclusion Statement Development and Evidence Grading

The collection, description, and synthesis of evidence are subsequently used by the DGAC subcommittee to develop a conclusion statement in response to the systematic review question. Conclusion statements are written in a clear and concise manner and include relevant information important for consideration, including a statement acknowledging general agreement among the studies on which the conclusion was based, and/or an explanation of any areas of disagreement. Per NEL protocol, conclusion statements are not to address areas outside of the body of evidence reviewed and are not intended to express implications. Drafting conclusion statements, as with the evidence description and synthesis, is an iterative process involving both DGAC subcommittee and NEL staff. The DGAC subcommittee's role is to ensure appropriate interpretation and communication of evidence, while the NEL staff's role is to review draft conclusions to ensure they met the protocol. If discussions throughout the evidence synthesis and drafting of conclusion statements necessitates clarifications or changes to the evidence portfolio, these are made by the NEL staff as appropriate.

Each conclusion statement is accompanied by a grade of the strength of the evidence supporting the conclusion; the grade is not applicable to individual studies. The grade is determined by the DGAC subcommittee according to specific criteria laid out by the NEL and based on five elements: internal validity, adequacy, consistency, impact, and generalizability.

1. Internal validity refers to the "likelihood that the reported effects are the true effects of the intervention/exposure and not over- or

underestimates resulting from bias due to study design or conduct" and is based on information gathered in completing the NEL BAT (USDA/HHS, 2016).

2. Adequacy of the evidence is determined based on the number of "studies overall, studies by independent research groups, studies with sample sizes that are sufficient to avoid type I and II errors, and participants overall" (USDA/HHS, 2016).
3. Consistency of the evidence is judged on three elements of the findings: "(1) direction, (2) size of effect/degree of association, and (3) statistical significance" (USDA/HHS, 2016).
4. Impact of the evidence is determined by: "(1) the directness with which the study designs examine the link between the intervention/exposure and outcome of interest in the systematic review question, (2) the statistical significance, and (3) the practical/clinical significance" (USDA/HHS, 2016).
5. Generalizability of the evidence to the U.S. population is considered with regard to the study samples and the intervention/exposure and outcomes studied.

For each of these five elements, the DGAC determines whether the overall body of evidence in each area is strong, moderate, or limited, or whether a grade is not assignable. Each DGAC subcommittee member evaluates the body of evidence and assigns a grade for each of those elements independently, and then differences are noted and discussed among the DGAC subcommittee members. Through discussion, the DGAC subcommittee arrives at a grade for the conclusion statement, reflective of its evaluation of the overall body of evidence as outlined in the NEL grading rubric. The grades used for conclusion statements also fall into one of these four categories: strong, moderate, limited, and grade not assignable (see Table 6-3). Draft and final conclusion statements and grades are presented at public meetings.

Step 6: Identification of Research Recommendations

Research recommendations are initially developed and drafted during the evidence description and synthesis step to reflect gaps and/or limitations in the body of evidence, but can be revised and updated to reflect the continued discussions concerning conclusions and grading of evidence before being finalized. Emerging topics in particular can be included in the *DGAC Scientific Report* with a rationale describing the need for additional research.

TABLE 6-3 Description of Grades for Conclusion Statements Used by the USDA Nutrition Evidence Library

Grade	Description
I—Strong	The conclusion statement is substantiated by a large, high-quality, and/or consistent body of evidence that directly addresses the question. There is a high level of certainty that the conclusion is generalizable to the population of interest, and it is unlikely to change if new evidence emerges.
II—Moderate	The conclusion statement is substantiated by sufficient evidence, but the level of certainty is restricted by limitations in the evidence, such as the amount of evidence available, inconsistencies in findings, or methodological or generalizability concerns. If new evidence emerges, there could be modifications to the conclusion statement.
III—Limited	The conclusion statement is substantiated by insufficient evidence, and the level of certainty is seriously restricted by limitations in the evidence, such as the amount of evidence available, inconsistencies in findings, or methodological or generalizability concerns. If new evidence emerges, there could likely be modifications to the conclusion statement.
IV—Grade not assignable	A conclusion statement cannot be drawn due to a lack of evidence or the availability of evidence that has serious methodological concerns.

SOURCE: USDA/HHS, 2016.

Availability and Accessibility of Systematic Reviews

Public availability of original systematic reviews is part of the NEL protocol. For example, the NEL systematic reviews are documented in their entirety and, following the completion of the review and the publication of the *DGAC Scientific Report*, are posted on the NEL website (NEL.gov) to promote transparency, accessibility, and reproducibility. Systematic reviews conducted for the DGAC are discussed at DGAC public meetings. Throughout the 2015 DGAC's deliberations, public comments were accepted, and comments about the systematic reviews under way were welcomed and reviewed by the 2015 DGAC. The completed evidence portfolio that is posted online following the publication of the *DGAC Scientific Report* includes

1. A conclusion statement;
2. A grade of the overall quality of evidence;
3. Key findings;
4. Research recommendations;

5. Evidence summaries giving the description and synthesis of the evidence along with the risk of bias assessment, references, and research recommendations;
6. An analytic framework, including the systematic review question(s); and
7. Search plan and results, including search parameters, selection criteria, and the final list of included and excluded articles, with brief explanations of reasons for exclusion (USDA/HHS, 2016).

The NEL staff drafts a technical abstract for each systematic review, which is posted on the NEL website along with the details of the full systematic review. The technical abstract is designed to provide key details of the systematic review in an easily accessible and standard format, similar in nature to a technical abstract prepared for peer-reviewed publications or scientific meetings, but longer and including more detail. Technical abstracts are reviewed by the DGAC subcommittee members before posting. Each technical abstract is titled with the systematic review question it describes, and includes five sections: background, conclusion statement, methods, findings, and discussion. Within these sections, key details of the systematic review are described, including the rationale and objective, data sources, study eligibility criteria, participants, interventions, study appraisal, synthesis methods, results of the systematic review and appraisal of the body of evidence along with the grade of the conclusion statement, and limitations and implications of key findings (USDA/HHS, 2016).

Approach to Non-DGAC Systematic Reviews

The NEL was created to support the DGAC, as well as conduct nutrition-related systematic reviews for federal partner agencies, such as those within USDA and HHS. As a result, the NEL has two separate protocols for conducting systematic reviews: one for DGAC-requested systematic reviews, and one for non-DGAC systematic reviews.[6] The two protocols have many similarities and use the same steps, but there are key differences.

The fundamental difference between the two protocols is that for DGAC-requested systematic reviews, the DGAC is the approver and "authors" the systematic review (USDA/HHS, 2017). In the protocol for non-DGAC systematic reviews, the NEL authors the work and relies on a technical expert collaborative to provide domain expertise. The technical

[6] In this discussion, details of the steps for the non-DGAC systematic review protocol were derived from two reports (USDA, 2012, 2014).

expert collaborative reviews key decisions and provides technical advice as needed (USDA, 2012, 2014). This difference drives much of the variation at the procedural level (e.g., key decisions made by the DGAC are instead made by the NEL).

Other key differences between the two protocols include the tools used. In Step 3, data extraction and risk of bias assessment, the protocol for DGAC systematic reviews employs the NEL BAT to evaluate bias (USDA/HHS, 2016). The non-DGAC systematic review protocol uses the Academy of Nutrition and Dietetics Research Design and Implementation Checklist to assess methodological rigor[7] (USDA, 2012, 2014). To conduct Step 5, developing conclusion statements and grading the evidence, different sets of criteria are used to evaluate strength of the body of evidence. The DGAC systematic review protocol employs the criteria of internal validity, adequacy, consistency, impact, and generalizability (USDA/HHS, 2016). The non-DGAC systematic review protocol, however, uses criteria adapted and validated by the Academy of Nutrition and Dietetics: quality, quantity, consistency, generalizability, and public health impact (USDA, 2012, 2014).

Evaluation of the NEL Original Systematic Review Process

Several organizations have developed guidance on conducting systematic reviews, including AHRQ, Cochrane, and the Institute of Medicine, which were all cited in the development of the NEL protocol (USDA/HHS, 2016). To assess the NEL process, the systematic review process from the *2015 DGAC Scientific Report* was outlined by this National Academies committee according to systematic review steps adapted from the report *Finding What Works in Health Care: Standards for Systematic Reviews* (IOM, 2011). These steps, as well as the roles of the NEL and DGAC in the process, are described in detail in Table 6-4. This National Academies committee reviewed each step in the systematic review process. Although the standards presented in Table 6-4 are aspirational and will likely not all be met in every systematic review, they do highlight several opportunities for improvement in the NEL de novo systematic review process, as discussed in the next section.

Findings

Original systematic reviews can help the DGAC answer questions regarding the relationship between diet and health if a synthesis of the

[7] The Academy of Nutrition and Dietetics' Research Design and Implementation Checklist uses the quality ratings of positive, neutral, or negative.

TABLE 6-4 Description of the Roles of the NEL and DGAC in the 2015 NEL Process Related to Conducting Systematic Reviews

Systematic Review Step	Role of NEL	Role of 2015 DGAC
1. Establish a team with appropriate expertise and experience to conduct the systematic review.	• The NEL was staffed by federal nutritionists and librarians with advanced degrees in nutrition, library science, or a related field who have expertise in systematic review methodology. o NEL staff was supported by abstractors, who were trained by NEL staff to review individual research articles included in NEL systematic reviews. Abstractors are nongovernmental professionals from across the United States with advanced degrees in nutrition or a related field.	• Subject-matter expertise varied across the 14-member DGAC; 3 consultants also provided additional expertise. • The DGAC divided into 5 subcommittees to conduct its review of evidence, including systematic reviews; 4–7 members were included on each subcommittee, based on expertise; 2 subcommittees added consultants to provide additional subject-matter expertise. (Working groups were similarly organized to address crosscutting topics later in the DGAC's deliberations.) • The DGAC balance plan specified that "prospective members of the advisory committee should have a broad knowledge of current scientific research in human nutrition; be familiar with the purpose, communication, and application of the Dietary Guidelines; be respected and published experts in their fields; represent a balance of viewpoints; and have a reputation for working well with others and being able to communicate clearly, both orally and in writing" (USDA/HHS, 2016).
1.1 Include expertise in pertinent clinical content areas.	• N/A	• Varies by DGAC; see 1
1.2 Include expertise in systematic review methods.	• Included on NEL staff	• Varies by DGAC; see 1

TABLE 6-4 Continued

Systematic Review Step	Role of NEL	Role of 2015 DGAC
1.3 Include expertise in searching for relevant evidence.	• Included on NEL staff	• Varies by DGAC; see 1
1.4 Include expertise in quantitative methods.	• Included on NEL staff	• Varies by DGAC; see 1
1.5 Include other expertise as appropriate.	• N/A	• Varies by DGAC; see 1
2. Manage biases and conflicts of interest (COIs) of the team conducting the systematic review.	(described below)	(described below)
2.1 Require each team member to disclose potential COI and professional or intellectual bias.	• Certain USDA employees hold positions requiring them to file the annual OGE Form 450, which includes disclosure of financial interests and other potential COIs as defined by 5 C.F.R. 2634.907. • NEL abstractors were required to disclose potential financial, intellectual, and professional COIs. Issues presented therein were discussed with the USDA Ethics Office, as needed (USDA/HHS, 2016).	• DGAC members were required to disclose potential financial COIs annually through OGE Form 450; professional and intellectual biases were noted to be considered in the selection of DGAC members but were not systematically collected (USDA/HHS, 2016). • Additional consideration of potential professional or intellectual bias was not noted to be conducted separately for each systematic review topic during the committee's review of the evidence.

continued

TABLE 6-4 Continued

Systematic Review Step	Role of NEL	Role of 2015 DGAC
2.2 Exclude individuals with a clear financial conflict.	• Federal employees are prohibited from participating in certain government matters when they have a financial COI, as required by 18 U.S.C. 208 and 5 C.F.R. 2640. • Abstractors who were deemed by federal staff to have potential conflicts or perceived conflicts that may unduly influence their contributions to the review project were not permitted to participate in that NEL review project (USDA/HHS, 2016).	• Individuals serving on the DGAC disclose potential COIs on the OGE Form 450 and are given tailored advice on potential remedies under 18 U.S.C. 208, including recusal, divestiture or waiver.
2.3 Exclude individuals whose professional or intellectual bias would diminish the credibility of the review in the eyes of the intended users.	• See 2.1 and 2.2	• See 2.1 and 2.2
3. Ensure user and stakeholder input as the review is designed and conducted.	Information about the design and conduct of systematic reviews was discussed during public meetings and made available at https://health.gov/dietaryguidelines.[a]	
3.1 Protect the independence of the review team to make the final decisions about the design, analysis, and reporting of the review.	Public comments about the systematic review design and conduct were received and reviewed by the 2015 DGAC.	

TABLE 6-4 Continued

Systematic Review Step	Role of NEL	Role of 2015 DGAC
4. Manage bias and COI for individuals providing input into the systematic review.	Public comments were accepted throughout the 2015 DGAC's deliberations, and submitters were required to provide their affiliation. Federal staff reviewed every comment and filtered out any duplicate, blank, or irrelevant comments.	
4.1 Require individuals to disclose potential COI and professional or intellectual bias.	Not reported.	
4.2 Exclude input from individuals whose COI or bias would diminish the credibility of the review in the eyes of the intended user.	Not reported.	
5. Formulate the topic for the systematic review.	(described below)	

continued

TABLE 6-4 Continued

Systematic Review Step	Role of NEL	Role of 2015 DGAC
5.1 Confirm the need for a new review.	• N/A	• DGAC used a set of criteria to aid in selecting topics that were within scope. • DGAC provided key information to use in identifying topics to be addressed (USDA/HHS, 2016). • Information collected during topic identification included a brief description of the topic and rationale that explained the importance of the topic, a description of the population, interventions/exposures, comparators, and outcomes of interest (PICO). • Factors considered in prioritizing topics for review included whether a review of the topic may result in the development of new recommendations, or a change or elaboration of existing recommendations; whether the topic represented an area of uncertainty or a knowledge gap, or an area of urgency for guidance; whether the topic addressed a dilemma in public health nutrition or addressed a common practice in public health nutrition for which no government guidance exists; or whether the topic had the potential to inform public health-oriented dietary guidance at the population/community level (HHS/USDA, 2013). • Topics were prioritized into tiers based on these criteria (USDA/HHS, 2016).

TABLE 6-4 Continued

Systematic Review Step	Role of NEL	Role of 2015 DGAC
5.2 Develop an analytic framework that clearly lays out the chain of logic that links the health intervention to the outcomes of interest and defines the key questions to be addressed by the systematic review.[b]	• N/A	• The DGAC developed an analytic framework, which served as a visual representation of the systematic review that defined and linked PICO elements as well as key confounders to consider. The framework illustrated the overall scope of the project, included definitions for key terms, and helped to ensure that all contributing elements in the causal chain would be examined and evaluated.
5.3 Use a standard format to articulate each question of interest.[b]	• Using key information collected during topic identification, federal staff assisted the DGAC with drafting systematic review questions using the PICO framework.	• Draft systematic reviews questions were refined using an iterative process between the DGAC and the NEL, which incorporated the various scientific perspectives of the DGAC (USDA/HHS, 2016).
5.4 State the rationale for each question.[b]	• Not reported.	• Not reported.
5.5 Refine each question based on user and stakeholder input.[b]	• N/A	• Public comments about topics were received and considered by the 2015 DGAC and made available publicly online.
6. Develop a systematic review protocol.	(described below)	(described below)
6.1 Describe the context and rationale for the review from both a decision-making and research perspective.	• See 5.1 and 5.2	• See 5.1 and 5.2

continued

TABLE 6-4 Continued

Systematic Review Step	Role of NEL	Role of 2015 DGAC
6.2 Describe the study screening and selection criteria (inclusion/ exclusion criteria).	• The NEL established a set of standard inclusion/exclusion criteria.[a]	• Objective inclusion and exclusion criteria were modified as needed by the DGAC to ensure the most relevant body of evidence was identified to answer the question and included in the search plan and results; criteria were presented during public meetings and posted publicly as part of DGAC presentations immediately after meeting and after the completion of the review (DGAC, 2014).
6.3 Describe precisely which outcome measures, time points, interventions, and comparison groups will be addressed.	• N/A	• Included as part of the analytic framework developed by the DGAC (see 5.2); frameworks were presented during public meetings and posted publicly as part of DGAC presentations immediately after the public meetings and after the completion of the review.

TABLE 6-4 Continued

Systematic Review Step	Role of NEL	Role of 2015 DGAC
6.4 Describe the search strategy for identifying relevant evidence.	• NEL librarian determined search terms, databases, and search refinements, which were documented in the search plan and results posted publicly after the completion of the review. • NEL librarian and analysts may conduct a duplication assessment to determine whether any existing high-quality systematic reviews and/or meta-analyses existed that address systematic review questions posed. • NEL librarian conducted the literature search to identify primary literature to include in the systematic review. • To optimize each search, NEL librarians peer reviewed each other's search strategies, as well as compared to indexing of similar searches (USDA/HHS, 2016).	• The DGAC provided subject/topic terminology as needed to assist in choosing an appropriate and comprehensive set of search terms (USDA/HHS, 2016). • After the NEL librarian peer reviewed and updated the search strategy, the DGAC reviewed the final search strategy.
6.5 Describe the procedures for study selection.	• Two NEL analysts independently screened articles at the title, abstract, and full-text levels. • Analysts compiled lists of included and excluded articles with rationale.	• After NEL analysts' independent screening, the DGAC was provided with the summary of the search strategy and the search results, including a list of included and excluded articles, for review, additional input, and approval.

continued

TABLE 6-4 Continued

Systematic Review Step	Role of NEL	Role of 2015 DGAC
6.6 Describe the data extraction strategy.	• Evidence abstractors extracted key data from each article included in a systematic review. • Evidence abstractors used a standard data extraction form, which served as a description of the extraction method. • NEL analysts reviewed extracted data for each study for quality control purposes.	• In advance of the data extraction step, the DGAC reviewed and approved the standard data extraction form.
6.7 Describe the process for identifying and resolving disagreement between researchers in study selection and data extraction decisions.	• Differences between the analyst and abstractor regarding data extraction or NEL Bias Assessment Tool responses were resolved, and a third-party consultation with an additional member of the federal staff was solicited when needed (USDA/HHS, 2016).	• N/A
6.8 Describe the approach to critically appraising individual studies.	• NEL evidence abstractors and analysts independently assessed the internal validity of each study using the NEL Bias Assessment Tool to determine whether any systematic error existed to either over- or under-estimate the results.	• N/A

TABLE 6-4 Continued

Systematic Review Step	Role of NEL	Role of 2015 DGAC
6.9 Describe the method for evaluating the body of evidence, including the quantitative and qualitative synthesis strategies.	• N/A	• Step 1: DGAC reviewed the extracted data and full-text manuscripts and independently answered objective probing questions designed to facilitate the DGAC's review and analysis of the evidence.
	• Step 2: An NEL analyst used DGAC input to draft (1) an evidence description that included an overview of the subject characteristics, interventions/exposures, outcomes examined, methodology used, and summary of study results; and (2) an evidence synthesis that included a summary of themes, an overview table, assessment of the body of evidence, and research recommendations.	• N/A
	• N/A	• Step 3: Input obtained from the DGAC's responses to the probing questions and the evidence synthesis was compiled by an NEL analyst and was used by the DGAC to develop a draft conclusion statement. • The DGAC reviewed the final draft synthesis and conclusion statement to ensure that its input was interpreted correctly, to solicit responses to clarifying questions, and to request feedback on the synthesis and conclusion statement. • Step 4: The DGAC evaluated and graded the body of evidence for each conclusion using the NEL grading rubric, which is based on five elements—internal validity, adequacy, consistency, impact, and generalizability.

continued

TABLE 6-4 Continued

Systematic Review Step	Role of NEL	Role of 2015 DGAC
6.10 Describe and justify any planned analyses of differential treatment effects according to patient subgroups, how an intervention is delivered, or how an outcome is measured.[b]	• N/A	• Population subgroups of interest were identified as part of the analytic framework developed by the DGAC (see 5.2); frameworks were presented during public meetings and posted publicly as part of DGAC presentations immediately after the public meetings and after the completion of the review. Subgroup analyses were described in the review of evidence.
6.11 Describe the proposed timetable for conducting the review.	• NEL reviews for the DGAC must take place within the time that the DGAC is active; other reviews can be conducted outside that 2-year period, but are not considered to be part of the DGAC review. They can be used by the DGAC as existing evidence (e.g., dietary patterns systematic review report).	• N/A
7. Submit the protocol for peer review.	The protocol for individual systematic reviews was not submitted for peer review.	
7.1 Provide a public comment period for the protocol and publicly report on disposition of comments.	A public comment period was not explicitly provided for each protocol. Public comments are accepted at any time and on any topic throughout the DGAC's review of the evidence.	

TABLE 6-4 Continued

Systematic Review Step	Role of NEL	Role of 2015 DGAC
8. Make the final protocol publicly available, and add any amendments to the protocol in a timely fashion.	The final protocol was posted on NEL.gov after completion of the review and publication of the DGAC report.	

NOTES: This table describes the NEL systematic review protocol as based on the 2015 DGAC process. The numbered systematic review steps are adapted from the Institute of Medicine report *Finding What Works in Health Care: Standards for Systematic Reviews*. The systematic review team was considered to include NEL staff, abstractors, and the DGAC members. DGAC members were not considered to be users/stakeholders. DGAC = 2015 Dietary Guidelines Advisory Committee; N/A = not applicable; NEL = Nutrition Evidence Library; OGE = Office of Government Ethics; PICO = population, intervention/exposure, comparator, and outcome of interest; USDA = U.S. Department of Agriculture.

[a] The NEL has established standard processes (e.g., inclusion and exclusion criteria) to help promote consistency across NEL reviews and to ensure that the evidence being considered in each systematic review is applicable to the U.S. population and relevant to public health- and nutrition-oriented policies and programs. These standard processes have been reviewed and informed by federal stakeholders to ensure policy relevance.

[b] This standard was adapted to apply to the NEL process.

SOURCES: DGAC, 2014; HHS/USDA, 2013; IOM, 2011; USDA/HHS, 2016.

evidence does not already exist. The utility of original systematic reviews depends on the availability of high-quality studies that are implemented appropriately to ensure impartiality of the reviews. The DGAC protocol could be better structured to support independence of NEL de novo systematic reviews.

The roles of the NEL staff and the DGAC are not clearly delineated and overlap at many steps of the systematic review protocol, potentially limiting the objectivity of results. For example, in evaluating the body of evidence, the DGAC's process for synthesizing evidence and drafting conclusion statements appears to be facilitated by the NEL staff (i.e., NEL staff develops probing questions for the DGAC's review of the evidence as well as compiles information received from the DGAC), but the statements are both "drafted" by the DGAC and then "reviewed" by the DGAC. The position of the DGAC as the driver of each step in the systematic review process, from the designing of the search strategy to the grading of the body of evidence, does not consistently promote an independent process. This National Academies committee's evaluation also identified the challenge of combining a systematic review process with the process for developing *DGA* recommendations, as best practices have shown that development of guidelines generally requires a more thorough separation of steps. While still allowing for the necessary iterations and communication between DGAC and NEL staff, this National Academies committee believes there is an opportunity to limit the overlap in roles and ensure the necessary expertise is included appropriately in each step by redesigning the process to clearly delineate the roles of both the DGAC and the NEL staff (see Chapter 4).

Because systematic reviews synthesize the evidence presented in individual studies, it is critical that the primary studies are of high quality. Nutrition studies present several methodological challenges, one in particular being self-reported dietary intake data. Because methods for acquiring dietary intake data vary and have the potential to introduce bias into the systematic review outcomes, they should be taken into account in the development of inclusion/exclusion criteria and appropriately managed in analyses whenever possible (see Box 4-4 for a discussion on using self-reported dietary intake data).

Throughout the entire process of conducting systematic reviews, it is unclear how and with what frequency NEL methods are updated. For example, since the NEL BAT was developed, other organizations have made several improvements in assessing the risk of bias in systematic reviews (Higgins and Green, 2011; Viswanathan et al., 2012). However, these updates have not yet been reflected in the NEL BAT. Additionally, while NEL de novo systematic reviews are publicly available, they are not peer reviewed. Maintaining up-to-date methods for conducting systematic reviews in a rapidly evolving field depends on collaboration with outside organizations and implementing ongoing training in best practices.

In addition, appropriately interpreting the results of systematic reviews, and subsequently integrating these results with other analyses, is an important element in developing conclusions. The interpretation of results and integration of analyses are subjective and require careful consideration. Whereas many steps are in place earlier in the NEL systematic review process to help identify potential limitations in the data available (e.g., inclusion/exclusion criteria, risk of bias assessment), it is unclear how these limitations are taken into account in the interpretation of results.

Conclusion

Overall, the NEL process for conducting original systematic reviews is thorough and adheres to several of the existing systematic review standards in the field. However, the overall protocol needs to be strengthened to improve the efficiency of the NEL process and minimize the introduction of bias. Clear delineation of the roles of individuals and groups involved at various steps in the NEL process are key to developing appropriate conclusions. The NEL ought to use the most appropriate, validated, and standardized methods whenever possible. Ensuring up-to-date methods are adopted and implemented in the NEL process depends on engaging in ongoing training and collaboration efforts with other organizations conducting systematic reviews, and could increase the usefulness of the NEL. Systematic reviews including observational studies in particular will need to be carefully evaluated in the interpretation of results and development of conclusions.

ASSESSMENT OF THE NEL PROCESS FOR UPDATING SYSTEMATIC REVIEWS

Because the NEL has only been used to support two editions of the *DGAC Scientific Report*, the only opportunity to update systematic reviews conducted previously by the NEL was in the 2015 DGAC. In one instance, the update combined two questions into one and expanded the terminology around the exposure of interest in the search to broaden the scope of the systematic review, while keeping the target population and outcomes the same. In the other instances, the same systematic review was repeated with updated search dates for the purpose of capturing articles published after the original systematic review was conducted. Updates of NEL systematic reviews were conducted and documented according to NEL de novo systematic review methods (HHS/USDA, 2015b). Methods for conducting an update to an existing systematic review not original to the NEL will be discussed in the assessment of existing systematic reviews, meta-analyses, and reports.

Findings

Systematic reviews can be updated to take into account new evidence since the last review was conducted. The NEL process for updating systematic reviews reflects the process for original systematic reviews, and the findings identified for conducting original systematic reviews apply also to the process for updating systematic reviews.

In the *2015 DGAC Scientific Report*, a clear explanation of why a decision was made to update or not update a systematic review was not publicly available. Updating systematic reviews can be done for a number of reasons and takes several forms (AHRQ, 2014; Garner et al., 2016; Higgins and Green, 2011). In some cases, such as abstracting new data or significantly adjusting the methods used, updating a systematic review can require more resources than conducting a de novo review. Reasons to update a systematic review could include any one or multiple of the following scenarios:

1. The systematic review question to be answered and the methods to be used remain unchanged, but the review does not include recently published studies on the topic. This gap requires adding recently published studies. This approach also assumes that either the results or the abstracted data from previous systematic reviews are available so that quantitative analyses could be performed, if needed.
2. If the systematic review question is changed (different from an existing systematic review), it may require abstracting new data from publications used in previous systematic reviews. An outcome of interest or metric may also change (e.g., measurement of dietary intake). In this case, a new search may or may not be needed.
3. Methods used in systematic reviews also evolve (e.g., grading of evidence, the use of different types of self-reported dietary data); adhering to the latest standards in performing an update sometimes requires using data abstracted from primary publications in a previous systematic review.

Conclusion

It was not clear why the 2015 DGAC chose to update some systematic reviews and not others. Updates of NEL systematic reviews generally ought to be conducted on a needs-based approach and in accordance with the NEL systematic review protocol for de novo systematic reviews. Regardless of the reason to update a systematic review, an update needs to consider all relevant research. Updating a systematic review may require collecting additional data or performing new analyses. As a result, newly published studies may be added or previously included studies may be excluded based on refined methods. This includes previously appraised research, because advances in knowledge about mechanisms of action, interactions of nutrients, or other factors that affect the outcome may reflect new understandings and could be integrated into a new conclusion statement.

Because new information and publications often drive updates, ongoing surveillance of literature is necessary to keep systematic reviews up to date and minimize duplication of efforts. Ongoing surveillance can also identify existing systematic reviews that may replace the need to conduct an update of a systematic review.

ASSESSMENT OF THE NEL PROCESS FOR USING EXISTING SYSTEMATIC REVIEWS, META-ANALYSES, AND REPORTS

Many groups around the world are now conducting systematic reviews, often on the same topic. Because systematic reviews require significant amounts of time, expertise, and costs to conduct, a search should be made to identify existing and ongoing systematic reviews before a new systematic review is undertaken. With limited resources, it would be advantageous to leverage existing systematic reviews, meta-analyses, and reports to minimize unnecessary replication of efforts and to share results with others.

However, existing systematic reviews may not fully address the question or population of interest, they may be outdated, or they may not meet current methodological standards. Furthermore, the quality of the systematic reviews—and hence their reliability—may vary. These concerns can make use of existing systematic reviews challenging but do not necessarily invalidate these systematic reviews. The concerns must be carefully analyzed and the challenges in using them understood. If a decision is made to proceed with using existing systematic reviews, documenting the rationale and explaining how any challenges are mitigated provides transparency. Documenting the reasons that existing systematic reviews have been assessed but not included will assist in reconciling potential differences in the results across different systematic reviews.

DGAC Approach to Using Existing Systematic Reviews, Meta-Analyses, and Reports

In addition to conducting original systematic reviews, the DGAC has used existing systematic reviews, meta-analyses, and reports to answer its questions. The 2015 DGAC was the first committee to develop and document a standardized process and criteria for including existing systematic reviews. The process paralleled several of the steps in the de novo NEL systematic review process.

Identifying Existing Systematic Reviews, Meta-Analyses, and Reports

As systematic review questions were developed and prioritized, the DGAC collaborated with the NEL to develop an analytic framework. At this point, before the literature search and screening begins, existing systematic reviews, meta-analyses, and reports may have been identified a priori by DGAC subcommittee members aware of current literature. The 2015 DGAC also requested literature and references on specific topics through public comments. If a report from an authoritative source was identified and met the criteria for inclusion, a literature search was still conducted according to NEL protocol to identify any additional reports on the topic. Existing reports may also have been identified during a duplication assessment in the early stages of the literature screening and selection process in preparation for a de novo systematic review (USDA/HHS, 2016). In all cases, the existing reports were required to meet the criteria for inclusion.

Criteria for Inclusion

Existing systematic reviews, meta-analyses, and reports were assessed by the NEL and the DGAC to determine if they met the predetermined inclusion/exclusion criteria. In some cases, federal DGAC support staff other than the NEL supported the DGAC in its review of existing systematic reviews, meta-analyses, and reports. The DGAC based its determination on four criteria: (1) the relevance to the systematic review question of interest, (2) the quality of the report, (3) the timeliness, and (4) reference overlap, if multiple systematic reviews were identified.

The relevance to the systematic review question was determined through comparison of the existing report to the established scope of the question outlined in the analytic framework, including PICO stipulations. Inclusion and exclusion criteria used in the existing report were also compared to those outlined for the question to judge relevance. For the 2015 DGAC, the methodological quality of the existing report was evaluated based on the AMSTAR tool, which considers 11 areas of methodological quality elements to assess.[8] In the AMSTAR tool, a systematic review receives 1 "point" for each item appropriately fulfilled, with a total score of 11 possible. To meet the inclusion criteria set by the DGAC in 2015, systematic reviews and/or meta-analyses must have scored 8 or higher (USDA/HHS, 2016). Timeliness of the systematic review was based on whether the date range set in the inclusion/exclusion criteria for the existing systematic review matched the date range set in the search strategy for the systematic review question of interest. In cases where multiple existing reports were identified, the references lists were examined for overlap. If individual studies overlap between system-

[8] These 11 criteria are (1) a priori research design established, (2) study selection and data extraction completed by two independent reviewers, (3) comprehensive review of literature conducted, (4) status of publication defined in inclusion criteria, (5) list of included and excluded studies provided, (6) characteristics of included studies provided, (7) scientific quality of included studies assessed and documented, (8) scientific quality of included studies considered in analysis and conclusions drawn, (9) appropriate methods applied for combining findings of studies, (10) assessment of the likelihood of publication bias included, and (11) conflict of interest in included studies and systematic review noted (Shea et al., 2007).

atic reviews, care was taken to ensure that the individual studies were not included multiple times, to reduce the potential for overestimating results (USDA/HHS, 2016).

Evidence Summary and Synthesis

If eligible for inclusion, a summary and synthesis of the evidence from existing reports was developed by federal DGAC support staff. In some cases, targeted questions may have been prepared by the federal staff to facilitate the DGAC members' identification of themes and key findings from the systematic reviews. The review of evidence specific to each systematic review question was outlined in the *2015 DGAC Scientific Report* (at the same level of detail as with original systematic reviews, including a conclusion statement and grade, implication statement, and summary of the review of evidence), and more detailed evidence descriptions were provided in appendixes to the *2015 DGAC Scientific Report* (HHS/USDA, 2015b). Although the information provided in the *2015 DGAC Scientific Report* varied slightly in the presentation and type of information for a particular systematic review question, at minimum, the report included an evidence portfolio with a summary table of included studies. For some systematic review questions, additional information such as the search strategy and analytic framework were included. Excluded studies, with briefly stated reasons for exclusion, were also provided as either a complete reference list of excluded studies or the number of excluded studies.

Historically, the DGAC has also considered existing authoritative reports published by federal agencies or leading scientific organizations in its evidence review. For these questions, an evidence portfolio was not provided, because the conclusions were drawn directly from published reports. For example, several questions in the *2015 DGAC Scientific Report* intended to address evidence on physical activity and health outcomes were based on conclusions from the *Physical Activity Guidelines Advisory Report, 2008*, and associated publications (HHS/USDA, 2015b).

Findings

Use of existing systematic reviews, meta-analyses, and reports may be beneficial, considering the significant time and resources needed to conduct original systematic reviews. Using existing systematic reviews also serves to limit the duplication of efforts across groups conducting systematic reviews. However, inclusion of existing systematic reviews, meta-analyses, and reports depends on their quality and relevance in relation to the specific topic and question that is being considered. As is the case for de novo systematic reviews, it is critical that the individual studies included in existing systematic reviews, meta-analyses, and reports are of high quality and adhere to standard methods.

Currently, the DGAC's criteria note that systematic reviews must achieve an AMSTAR score of 8 or higher to be included; however, limitations to the AMSTAR tool have been identified (Burda et al., 2016; Faggion, 2015; Wegewitz et al., 2016), and this measure alone is not sufficient to determine the quality of a systematic review. As methods continue to advance, the DGAC criteria will need to adjust accordingly.

Within the DGAC's stated criteria of inclusion, there are additional considerations, some of which are inherent to comparing reports, and others are specific challenges that may result in inabilities to use the existing systematic reviews as is. The assessment of published systematic reviews is based on reported information, which can vary widely across systematic reviews. A common challenge in using existing systematic reviews and relying on reported information is not having the necessary information to allow independent verification of the validity of the analyses and conclusions. Without the abilities to verify, the user of an existing systematic review has to trust the veracity of the reported information. Alternatively, the user may decide to use the existing systematic review as a framework and abstract only sufficient information from the original studies to carry out the necessary independent assessment.

Registration of the systematic review protocol on the PROSPERO website may provide additional information to assess whether the systematic review adhered to its original intent and methods. Archiving of data in websites such as the Systematic Review Data Repository provide opportunities for readers to assess the comprehensiveness and accuracy of the abstracted data used in systematic reviews. Although resources such as the Systematic Review Data Repository could increase transparency within the NEL process, their use is not required across organizations conducting systematic reviews, and many published systematic reviews may not have done so.

A more challenging problem occurs if disagreements in results and conclusions occur among multiple systematic reviews. The reason for discrepancy may sometimes be apparent, such as the obvious differences in the eligibility criteria or large differences in publication date and hence studies included. Discrepancies caused by subtle differences in the eligibility criteria or how such criteria were operationalized may be difficult to ascertain.

Missing data in the original systematic review may lead to an inability to include the systematic review, or the systematic review team may need to abstract additional information not reported by the original team that conducted the systematic review. It is difficult to know how the other team operationalized eligibility criteria, even if the written criteria appear the same. Different methods used to assess the limitations of primary studies and grade the strength of evidence can also present challenges.

In some cases, the NEL staff, in determining inclusion of an existing systematic review, may be able to simply perform a new literature search to bring the existing review up to date, if they determined that the data abstraction and analyses performed by the original authors were accurate, and their interpretations were correct. In these cases, the NEL and DGAC would need to ensure data abstraction and interpretation were harmonized with the NEL protocol. Even if an existing systematic review is found not to be completely suitable because of the nature of the question(s) asked, the list of studies identified may still be helpful in conducting a new systematic review.

Conclusion

In summary, use of existing systematic reviews, meta-analyses, and authoritative reports from leading organizations is generally appropriate and encouraged by this National Academies committee, with the understanding that they ought to be relevant, timely, and of high quality. Efficiency and use of time and resources must be weighed carefully in using an existing systematic review compared to conducting a de novo review (Smith et al., 2011; Whitlock et al., 2008). However, opportunities exist to strengthen the current method of identifying existing systematic reviews, meta-analyses, and reports. Ongoing surveillance of the literature can serve to identify existing systematic reviews while maximizing resources. Surveillance can also help identify authoritative reports for use by the DGAC. There are also opportunities to leverage the Systematic Review Data Repository at AHRQ to further enhance the value and usefulness of the NEL to the nutrition research community. All systematic reviews and reports ought to meet the criteria for inclusion specified in the NEL protocol, with consideration for appropriate methods in cases of missing and unreported data.

EVALUATION OF METHODOLOGY AND USE OF FOOD PATTERN MODELING

Since the *1990 DGA Policy Report*, specific food-intake guidance has been provided to help the public meet nutrient needs while moderating intake of other dietary constituents. Such guidance has been presented as a single food guide or multiple eating patterns (the USDA food patterns were substantially revised and formally described beginning in the *2005 DGAC Scientific Report*), but the intention has remained the same: translate nutritional recommendations into food intake recommendations that take account of the totality of the diet. In each instance, USDA has conducted food pattern modeling to derive this guidance for the DGAC.

Questions Food Pattern Modeling Is Intended to Address

Food pattern modeling, which assesses the nutrient content of various possible eating patterns based on typical choices within food groups, can be used to address a range of specific questions (see Appendix C). But the overarching question it seeks to answer is, "How well do varying combinations and amounts of food groups meet the Dietary Reference Intakes and potential recommendations in the *DGA*?" (Britten et al., 2006a,b). This is an important issue, given the myriad nutritional profiles of basic foods and the complex array of constraints involved in achieving nutritional adequacy while moderating consumption of energy and other dietary constituents. In effect, food pattern modeling shows how diets *could* be developed to meet those constraints. Three different patterns developed by USDA were featured in the *2015–2020 DGA Policy Report*—"Healthy US-Style," "Healthy Mediterranean-Style," and "Healthy Vegetarian"—as "examples of healthy eating patterns that can be adapted based on cultural and personal preferences" (HHS/USDA, 2015a). The Dietary Approaches to Stop Hypertension (DASH) dietary pattern is also mentioned in the *2015–2020 DGA Policy Report* as an "example of a healthy eating pattern . . . [with] . . . many of the same characteristics as the Healthy US-Style Eating Pattern" (HHS/USDA, 2015a). DASH was not derived via food pattern modeling; it was developed for a randomized controlled clinical trial to study the effect of that diet on cardiovascular risk factors.

Current Methods Used to Derive Evidence: Steps in Process

Food pattern modeling that both informs and reflects the *DGA* recommendations has been an iterative process, at times developed concurrently with the *DGA*, with input from both the DGAC and federal staff (Britten et al., 2006a). For the 2015 DGAC, USDA staff from the Center for Nutrition Policy and Promotion were designated by their leadership to work on food pattern modeling. They worked extensively with the DGAC in addressing possible modifications to the patterns through their support of DGAC committees. However, the DGAC and federal staff had unique roles in the process (see Figure 6-1).

The methods USDA employed to conduct the food pattern modeling required inherent assumptions in addressing the questions in Appendix C (Britten et al., 2006b). The first was that each specific question referred to the "total" rather than a "foundation" diet. Unlike other approaches to food

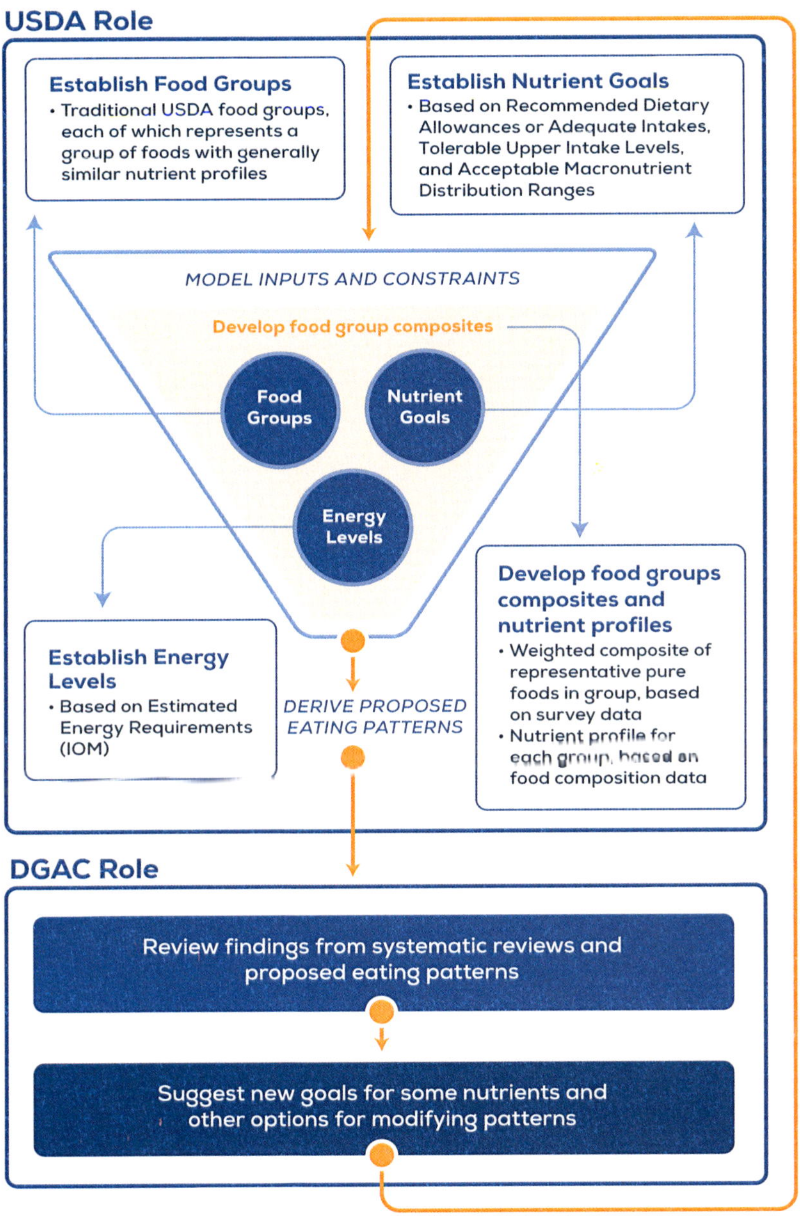

FIGURE 6-1 The roles of USDA staff and the DGAC in the current process for food pattern modeling.

NOTES: The traditional USDA food groups are vegetables, fruits, grains, dairy, protein foods, oils, and calories for other uses. DGAC = Dietary Guidelines Advisory Committee; IOM = Institute of Medicine; USDA = U.S. Department of Agriculture.

guidance that focus only on major nutrient-bearing food groups (i.e., the foundation), the food pattern modeling accounted for the totality of the diet (i.e., the entire energy allotment). The second assumption was that nutrient values associated with each pattern were based on typical food choices, but in their most nutrient-dense form. That is, by design, the nutrient profile associated with each food group corresponded to average nutrient values associated with a population-weighted mix of pure foods in that group.

The exact procedure involved in food pattern modeling depends on the specific question being addressed, but the general process is outlined in Figure 6-1 and described below.

Step 1: Establish Energy Levels

The first step in formulating the food patterns is establishing the set of energy levels for which discrete patterns will be developed. Energy requirements vary widely by gender, age, height, weight, and activity level (IOM, 2000), and the patterns that result from the modeling must cover the needs of nearly everyone in the population. Consequently, establishing the appropriate range of energy levels is key to the exercise. Using the IOM's formulas for calculating Estimated Energy Requirements (EERs) (IOM, 2005) for sedentary individuals, USDA determined that 1,000 to 3,200 kcal is an appropriate range. EERs represent the average energy intake predicted to maintain energy balance. USDA divided that range into 200-kcal increments, identified age/gender groups associated with each energy level, and then developed distinct patterns for each (Britten et al., 2006b).

Step 2: Establish Nutrient Goals

The second step in creating the patterns is to set the goals for a range of micro- and macronutrients at each energy level, based on the age/gender group(s) corresponding to that level. Goals for nutritional adequacy in the food patterns are based on the IOM's Recommended Dietary Allowances (RDAs) or Adequate Intakes (AIs), rather than the Estimated Average Requirements (EARs), because the patterns are intended to serve as guides for individuals in planning their intakes (see Appendix E). Patterns can exceed the RDA or the AI for some nutrients to meet the goals for others if they do not exceed the Tolerable Upper Intake Level (UL). For example, the goal for total fiber is set at 14 gm per 1,000 kcal, the formula used to set the AI. Moderation goals for nutrients that tend to be overconsumed are set at the Acceptable Macronutrient Distribution Range (AMDR) for the macronutrients and at less than the UL for sodium.

Step 3: Establish Food Groups

The next step is establishing the food groups, which form the "building blocks" of the pattern. Although the names have varied, five major food groups have formed the basis of USDA's food guidance for the past several decades: fruits, vegetables, grains, protein foods, and dairy. In addition, subgroups within several of these groups are constructed to target specific choices. For example, the grains group is subdivided into whole and refined grains, to encourage more frequent consumption of whole grains. In effect, dividing the group allows the modeling to change one subgroup more, less, or in a different direction than another, as needed to reach nutritional goals. The current list of food groups and subgroups in USDA's Healthy US-Style Eating Pattern and Healthy Mediterranean-Style Pattern is shown in Box 6-1; more discrete subgroups in the protein foods group (eggs, legumes, soy products, nuts, and seeds) replace meat, poultry, and eggs in the Healthy Vegetarian Eating Pattern.

BOX 6-1
Food Groups and Subgroups in USDA's Healthy Eating Patterns

- Vegetables
  - Dark-green vegetables
  - Red and orange vegetables
  - Legumes (beans and peas)
  - Starchy vegetables
  - Other vegetables
- Fruits
- Grains
  - Whole grains
  - Refined grains
- Dairy
- Protein foods
  - Seafood
  - Meat, poultry, eggs
  - Nuts, seeds, soy products
- Oils
- Calories for other uses

NOTE: More discrete subgroups in the protein foods group (eggs, legumes, soy products, nuts, and seeds) replace meat, poultry, and seafood in the Healthy Vegetarian Eating Pattern.
SOURCE: USDA, 2015.

Step 4: Develop Food Groups Composites and Nutrient Profiles

Once the food groups have been established, modelers identified the nutrient contributions from standard amounts of each to estimate the nutrient totals associated with varying quantities of the food groups and subgroups. A nutrient profile for each group and subgroup was determined by developing a weighted composite of representative foods from each group. These representative foods, and the weight each one receives in the composite, were determined based on national surveys. For example, potatoes made up most of the starchy vegetables composite because they represented the largest share of all starchy vegetables consumed; corn and peas were also included, but in lesser amounts. However, there was one important qualification: all candidate foods were in their leanest form, prepared without the addition of fat, oil, or sugar (Marcoe et al., 2006). For example, the dairy group was represented by fat-free fluid milk. This means, for example, if someone chooses low-fat vanilla yogurt instead of fat-free, any energy ascribed to the fat and added sugars must come from the relatively small "calories for other uses" allowance.

Step 5: Model Inputs and Constraints

The last step in deriving the proposed patterns—modeling the inputs and constraints to establish the amounts from each food group to achieve nutrient targets—is done iteratively to determine the best fit. The resulting patterns can also be compared to estimates of usual intakes of various foods from a recent National Health and Nutrition Examination Survey or other population surveys (see "Descriptive Data Analyses: Evaluation of Methodology and Use" beginning on page 180).

Review of Food Pattern Modeling

The methods and results of the food pattern modeling have been described in detail and peer reviewed via a number of manuscripts in the nutrition literature (Britten et al., 2006a,b; Marcoe et al., 2006). However, there is a difference between the kind of review a manuscript receives describing something that has already been completed and an invited review by outside experts to critique and advance a methodological process. Food pattern modeling could benefit from such a review.

Role of the DGAC in Food Pattern Modeling

The other steps shown in Figure 6-1 are initiated by the DGAC (i.e., review findings from systematic reviews along with proposed eating patterns and suggesting new goals for some nutrients and other options for modifying patterns), but USDA works in close collaboration with the DGAC to complete them. These steps may also be conducted iteratively, as they relate to evaluating the patterns and their possible modifications, based on the DGAC's assessment of findings from the systematic reviews and other descriptive data analyses. Many of the questions shown in Appendix C involve these steps. For example, identifying the amount of any nutrient in the overall pattern that is contributed by each of the food groups is done to determine each group's significance to the overall pattern and the extent to which it helps attain appropriate levels of nutrients of concern. If a nutrient tends to be limiting, options can be explored for modifying the patterns, based on which food groups are good sources and accompanying data on usual intakes of those food groups. The preset energy levels infer a "zero-sum game," so increases of one food group necessarily call for decreases in something else.

Findings

Modeling in general can be helpful in examining complex systems, and the food pattern modeling conducted by USDA has tremendous potential for showing the simultaneous effects of altering food intake patterns, given certain assumptions. Food pattern modeling is dependent on the accuracy of the assumptions, which need to be presented transparently to facilitate broad understanding of the methodology. These assumptions could be better structured to use the most current evidence available and be flexible enough to adjust to reflect new research, if necessary.

The preset energy levels and nutritional goals that serve as constraints in the modeling exercise are drawn from the relevant IOM standards (IOM, 2000). Energy levels designated to correspond to each sex and age group assume a sedentary activity level—rather than erring on the side of a larger energy allowance (which would make meeting nutrient needs easier)—because Americans tend to be both sedentary and overweight. The use of the RDA when available, and the AI otherwise, is fitting for guidance aimed at individuals rather than groups (IOM, 2000; Murphy and Barr, 2006). However, when comparing population usual intakes to proposed food group recommendations, it is important to note that the standards on which food group recommendations are based are intended to cover the requirements of nearly everyone in the population and so are likely higher than most people's needs. This is an important caveat because when recommendations are set to ensure the adequacy of almost everyone, as in this case, subsequent analyses examining, for example, whether Americans meet the recommendations, does not necessarily mean that most Americans are eating inadequate diets relative to their nutrient needs. In the long term, systems modeling may help identify if different recommendations are necessary for different groups or individuals and the potential effect of broader versus more tailored recommendations.

To date, a relatively limited set of food groupings has been used in the modeling. These groupings are defined based on nutrient content and their traditional place in the American diet. For example, the dairy group has always had a place in USDA guidance, because foods in that group are both *rich* sources of calcium (supplying a high amount per 100 gm of the food) and *important* sources (serving as a major contributor in U.S. diets) (Hoy and Goldman, 2014). However, some subcultures do not include dairy foods in their cuisine, and other segments of the population are lactose intolerant or allergic to dairy proteins. Recent iterations of USDA eating patterns have allowed soy beverages to substitute for animal milk, but that does not entirely address the mismatch between the guidance and the food and beverage preferences of many individuals.

The output of the food pattern modeling is in terms of the total daily quantity of foods from each group. The alternative would be to recommend a specific number of daily servings of a particular size, but the term *servings* can be confusing because portion sizes vary widely. Quantities for disparate foods within the groups are standardized with the use of "equivalents." For example, in the grain group, a half cup of cooked rice and one slice of bread are both considered to equal one ounce equivalent of grains.

Another issue is the lack of clarity regarding whether certain food groups and their amounts are *necessary*, or just *sufficient*, to achieve the modeling goals. Considering the example previously mentioned with dairy, it is not clear whether there is any other way to meet energy and calcium goals than by the inclusion of the recommended amounts of dairy foods. Another example is the vegetable subgroups: dark-green, red and orange, and legumes are undoubtedly targeted because they provide nutrients typically lacking in diets, but the question remains: are the starchy and other vegetables necessary (e.g., could the targeted subgroups alone supply all the vegetables)? Likewise, why are meats, poultry, and eggs all combined in one protein foods subgroup, given their differing nutrient profiles? It seems the idea of a food group's traditional role in the American diet may serve as an underlying constraint on the modeling, and a greater array of food group combinations and amounts may be possible that would meet energy and nutrient goals if that constraint were lifted. Again, by representing the pathways between different types of food and the resulting diet and then nutritional intake, systems models can show what may occur with various changes and replacements (e.g., what would happen if different foods were replaced by others?). Conducting a range of sensitivity analyses could provide insight into these relationships.

Employing and modeling different standards of "typical consumption"—operationalized by composite nutrient profiles weighted to reflect population averages—are critical, as they help evaluate what the population's average nutrient intake would be if they followed the recommendations under varying circumstances. The approach taken by DGAC is in contrast with others that rely on especially nutrient-dense foods (such as salmon, apricots, or almonds), which might result in insufficient nutrient intakes when the patterns are put into practice with more typically consumed foods. However, the *range* of expected nutrient intakes, as well as the *average*, could be obtained if the variability in intakes were accounted for. As an example, the composite nutrient profile for fruits is weighted toward orange juice, because it is a major fruit source in the population, and yet not everyone consumes orange juice. It would be helpful to perform some sensitivity analyses to see how dependent the estimated nutrient totals are to the inclusion of orange juice. It also might be useful to have separate composites for different age and sex groups if choices within the food groups vary by those demographics. Finally, typical consumption is inferred for choices within, not among, food groups because some food groups, although rarely consumed, are necessary to achieve nutrient adequacy.

As mentioned previously, although foods selected to represent the nutrient profile of each group are based on typical consumption, they are also in their leanest form, prepared without the addition of fat, oil, or added sugar. This approach seems intuitively contradictory because Americans typically eat foods with an overabundance of such additions; nonetheless, there is justification to examine potential patterns this way. Specifically, this prescription is followed precisely so the modelers can determine how much fat, oil, and sugars can be added to the diet. In other words, the purest forms of foods from nutrient-bearing food groups are assumed at the outset, to see how much of the energy allotment they alone require. A key result of the food pattern modeling is demonstrating there is a very small allowance for discretionary calories when trying to meet nutrient goals within energy levels appropriate for most Americans. In effect food modeling was used to set limits on substances such as fat, oil, and sugars rather than using a physiologic or metabolic end point. Systems models can account for the different additions and modifications (e.g., additives, cooking styles, preparation methods) that may occur to food prior to their consumption.

As defensible as it is to construct the patterns with the leanest, no-sugar-added form of all foods, this raises a key point regarding translation of the patterns. The most recent version of the *DGA* included some instruction regarding this point, in a figure titled "Hidden Components in Eating Patterns," but it is not at all clear whether consumers understand these distinctions. Obviously, if the recommended food group amounts were followed, but with foods in their usual forms, and additional discretionary calories were added, the total energy in the patterns would exceed the designated energy level. Alternatively, perhaps other assumptions could be made in the modeling to incorporate foods as consumed (such as including the saturated fat and sodium from cheese in the dairy composite, in proportion to its consumption).

A similar issue arises with sodium. Most representative foods in the composites are in a no-salt-added form; exceptions include bread (not low-sodium) and a small amount of ham in the meat composite. The relatively limited inclusion of foods containing salt and other sources of sodium results in patterns that approximate the UL without the addition of salt at the table, which is instructive regarding the austerity of the sodium UL.

Conclusion

In summary, the current process for food pattern modeling and its use in informing the DGAC review of the evidence is generally well designed for the questions it is intended to answer. The inputs, constraints, assumptions, and goals are all documented, and standard state-of-the-art data inputs are used. However, enhancements to the process could allow food pattern modeling to respond to a broader range of research questions, increasing its usefulness to the general population. Proposed enhancements include moving toward systems modeling, incorporating other factors and mechanisms that may affect the food composition and choice, further breaking down and representing the heterogeneity of the population and their behaviors, establishing more and different tailored scenarios, and conducting sensitivity analyses to determine how critical various food groups are as well as other key drivers. Sensitivity analyses can also help determine how robust the findings are to the inherent variability in food intakes and composition, and the resulting effect under a wider range of circumstances.

DESCRIPTIVE DATA ANALYSES: EVALUATION OF METHODOLOGY AND USE

Other types of questions that the DGAC is interested in answering are questions of prevalence, trends, and population-level food intake (see Table 6-1 and Appendix C), which are best answered with descriptive data. Previous DGACs have used national data to guide information regarding dietary, nutritional, and health status of the U.S. population. USDA and HHS staff with access to the data and expertise to conduct analyses have assisted in preparing these descriptive data analyses for the DGAC. Following the 2015 *DGA* cycle, these federal staff were collectively referred to as the Data Analysis Team (DAT). The post-hoc development of the DAT intends to improve efficiency regarding procurement and analyses of data requests of the DGAC. Aside from accessibility to appropriate data and willingness to assist the DGAC, no specific criteria for membership or inclusion on the DAT have been noted. The data were made publicly available through online access and inclusion in the *2015 DGAC Scientific Report*'s references and appendixes. Different from the questions completed by the NEL systematic reviews, the questions addressed using descriptive data analyses did not go through a grading rubric and were not graded. The DGAC acknowledged this issue by taking the "strengths and limitations of data analyses into account in formulating conclusion statements" (HHS/USDA, 2015b).

Questions That Descriptive Data Analyses Are Intended to Address

Descriptive data analyses are important with regard to providing information about the current status and trends in food and nutrient intakes among the population of the United States. Such information helped the DGAC evaluate adequacy of nutrient intake to determine whether there were "nutrients of concern" that may have been under- or overconsumed, as well as to indicate whether consumption should increase or decrease according to population consumption patterns (see Chapter 7 for additional information on determining nutrients of concern). The nutrient intake data provided information to determine whether nutrient intake of the U.S. population met the Dietary Reference Intakes (DRIs) recommendations. Data reporting the prevalence of diet-related diseases and conditions in the U.S. population aided the DGAC in its determination of the scope of current dietary problems. The specific questions addressed by these descriptive data analyses are outlined in Appendix C.

Sources of Descriptive Data and Methods Used by the 2015 DGAC

Whereas most of the analyses used data collected as part of NHANES, other important data sources were used by the 2015 DGAC, including government and nongovernment sources. These included the National Health Interview Survey and the 2014 report of the American Heart Association (HHS/USDA, 2015b) among others, as shown in Table 6-5.

A number of methods were used in the 2015 DGAC's assessment of available surveillance data to describe dietary and health status. Although stepwise descriptions of each analysis conducted to inform the

TABLE 6-5 Summary of Data Sources Used by the 2015 DGAC for Descriptive Data Analyses

Data Source	Use in 2015 DGAC
AHA statistics	• Prevalence of cardiovascular disease, stroke
NHANES	• Nutrient intake • Food group intake • Nutrient density by point of purchase and location of consumption • Selected eating behaviors • Selected biochemical indicators of diet and nutrition in the U.S. population • Prevalence of health conditions and trends, including body weight status, lipid profiles, high blood pressure, and diabetes
NHIS	• Prevalence of health conditions and trends (supplemental)
SEARCH Study	• Prevalence of diabetes
SEER	• Prevalence of selected cancers
USDA-ARS NND	• Food composition data[a]

NOTE: AHA = American Heart Association; NHANES = National Health and Nutrition Examination Survey; NHIS = National Health Interview Survey; SEARCH Study = SEARCH for Diabetes in Youth study; SEER = National Cancer Institute's Surveillance, Epidemiology, and End Results Program; USDA-ARS NND = U.S. Department of Agriculture's Agricultural Research Service National Nutrient Database for Standard Reference, Release 27.

[a] Includes data on energy and selected nutrients.

SOURCE: HHS/USDA, 2015b.

2015 DGAC Scientific Report were not available, the sources of data were included in the DGAC's description of the evidence (HHS/USDA, 2015b). The 2015 DGAC drew all dietary intake data from NHANES What We Eat in America (WWEIA), which offers detailed food intake and behavior information, as well as national- and subgroup-level estimates of usual dietary intakes.

NHANES WWEIA uses the interviewer-administered 24-hour dietary recall, which captures detailed dietary information for the past 24 hours through a verbal interview with participants. The 24-hour dietary recall method can provide rich detail about foods consumed. Although it measures intake only on a given day, and can be used to assess the mean intake for a population group, multiple 24-hour recalls for at least a representative subsample of individuals are required to estimate the distribution of usual intake for a population. Two recalls were collected for most individuals in WWEIA. The statistical method used by the DAT to estimate the distributions of usual nutrient and food intakes in a population was developed by scientists within NCI; thus, the method is colloquially and broadly referred to as the "NCI [National Cancer Institute] method" (NCI, 2015; Tooze et al., 2006).

Findings

This National Academies committee reviewed the approach of the DGAC, in collaboration with relevant federal partners (the DAT). The analytic approach used in determining the proportion of the population that is inadequate or at risk of adverse health effects owing to excess consumption adheres to the recommendations by the DRI committee on diet assessment, including the collection of multiple 24-hour dietary recalls, estimation of usual intake distributions, and comparisons of EARs to those distributions.

Another key element in the development of the guidelines is the availability of current data for use by the DGAC. This depends on both the timely release of data as well as timely analysis by the DAT. The descriptive data analyses used by the DGAC provide important inputs at the outset of the DGAC's review of evidence, including current prevalence of disease, trends, and population nutrient intakes, to inform further analyses and inform the identification of nutrients of concern. However, in the current process, these analyses are not initiated until the convening of the DGAC. Preparing these descriptive analyses in advance could maximize the DGAC's time. However, one caveat is that the most current data should be used by the DGAC, so any significant updates to datasets released after the initial analyses would need to be integrated throughout the DGAC's process. Additionally, recognizing that available population subgroup data may not fully represent the diversity of the U.S. population, exploring options to expand these data could be beneficial.

In reviewing descriptive data analyses conducted to inform past DGACs by various federal agencies and offices based on availability and relevance, this National Academies committee sees the introduction of the DAT as an opportunity for improving reporting of data analyses and centralizing efforts. For example, a central Web-based location that includes links to all the data analyses would be useful in increasing transparency and comparability of descriptive data analyses across *DGA* cycles.

This National Academies committee recognizes that data analyses depend on the availability of current and high-quality data collection efforts (e.g., surveillance data), and that advancements in the methods of data collection at the population and subgroup levels can also lead to improvements in the understanding of population health and disease prevalence and trends.

Conclusion

Overall, this National Academies committee found that the descriptive data analyses being conducted are appropriate to answer the questions proposed by the DGAC, and the availability of current and high-quality data continues to contribute to the most accurate analyses possible. Timely access to results of descriptive data analyses could maximize the DGAC's time and have important and lasting benefits for the *DGA* to affect changes in population health.

QUALITY OF DIETARY DATA ACROSS ALL TYPES OF EVIDENCE

Dietary intake data are central to the development of dietary guidelines, and form the basis of most studies examined in the systematic evidence-based reviews and analyses of food pattern modeling and consumption patterns of the population. The nutrition field has relied on respondent self-report as a means of assessing dietary intake to capture the totality of the diet. However, substantial limitations exist.

Regarding self-report, one of the limitations is measurement error, or the difference between the true value of a parameter of interest and the value obtained through assessment. There are two main types of measurement error: random and systematic. Random error occurs when measures scatter randomly around the true value. In dietary research, day-to-day variation in intakes is an example of this type of error. In descriptive research, random error does not affect the mean but leads to wider distributions and an overestimation of tail probabilities; in examining relationships, random error leads to attenuation and loss of power. Systematic error, or bias, occurs when measures tend to deviate from truth in the same direction; the widespread tendency to underreport intakes is an example of bias. Differential bias, such as the tendency toward greater underreporting among persons with obesity relative to other individuals, is particularly problematic because it confounds relationships between diet and health. In descriptive research, systematic error leads to inaccurate estimates of both the mean and the distribution. In examining associations, relationships can be either exaggerated or attenuated, depending on the source of the bias, and loss of power can result.

Different methods of collecting self-report dietary intake data exhibit varying degrees of each type of measurement error (NCI, 2017). Dietary recalls, which form the foundation of population dietary monitoring studies such as the NHANES WWEIA, generally exhibit more within-person random error because they are conducted on a 24-hour basis. Food frequency questionnaires, which have been used in most epidemiologic cohort studies, display relatively more bias.

Many researchers have described the effects of measurement error and what steps can be taken to address it, such as statistical adjustment and data cleaning methods that exclude implausible data (Freedman et al., 2011, 2017; Goldberg et al., 1991; Huang et al., 2005; Prentice and Huang, 2011; Tooze et al., 2010). Random within-person error can be corrected with repeat administrations and statistical modeling, and it is therefore generally less problematic than bias. Systematic error cannot be eliminated by repeated measures, but its effects can be addressed with the use of reference measures, such as biomarkers or a less biased instrument, on at least a subsample of individuals (NCI, 2017). Methods are continually being developed to address both types of error more effectively.

CONCLUSION

The types of analyses used in the *DGAC Scientific Report* include original systematic reviews; existing systematic reviews, meta-analyses, and reports; food pattern modeling; and descriptive data analyses. All types of analyses will continue to provide important information in the *DGA* going forward, and they need to be based on validated, standardized, and up-to-date methods and processes.

The NEL systematic review process overall is thorough and based on rigorous scientific standards. However, this National Academies committee identified opportunities for improvement in several areas where the NEL can be aligned with best practices. These areas include (1) a clear delineation of roles of the Dietary Guidelines Scientific Advisory Committee (DGSAC) and the NEL, (2) training for NEL staff, (3) collaboration with other systematic review groups, and (4) supportive infrastructure to keep NEL processes up to date. Additionally, ongoing surveillance of existing systematic reviews, meta-analyses, and reports can allow for less duplication of efforts and ensure outdated systematic reviews are updated and existing systematic reviews are used whenever possible. In using existing systematic reviews, the relevance, timeliness, and quality of the systematic review should be carefully considered according to NEL protocol and methodological standards.

Food pattern modeling and descriptive data analyses both provide unique and important inputs into the *DGA* process and could be improved with advanced and standardized methods. The current process for food pattern modeling operates within several assumptions, some of which are necessary and some of which can be updated to improve outcomes. Advancing methodology in the food pattern modeling process to account for variability in eating patterns could improve outcomes and increase the usefulness of the USDA food patterns. Conducting some descriptive data analyses and initial food pattern modeling in advance of the DGAC's convening, depending on the availability of current and high-quality data, could maximize time and increase efficiency of the *DGA* process.

REFERENCES

AHRQ (Agency for Healthcare Research and Quality). 2014. *Methods guide for effectiveness and comparative effectiveness reviews*. AHRQ Publication No. 10(14)-EHC063-EF.

Britten, P., J. Lyon, C. M. Weaver, P. M. Kris-Etherton, T. A. Nicklas, J. A. Weber, and C. A. Davis. 2006a. MyPyramid food intake pattern modeling for the Dietary Guidelines Advisory Committee. *Journal of Nutrition Education and Behavior* 38(Suppl 6):S143-S152.

Britten, P., K. Marcoe, S. Yamini, and C. Davis. 2006b. Development of food intake patterns for the MyPyramid food guidance system. *Journal of Nutrition Education and Behavior* 38(Suppl 6):S78-S92.

Burda, B. U., H. K. Holmer, and S. L. Norris. 2016. Limitations of a measurement tool to assess systematic reviews (AMSTAR) and suggestions for improvement. *Systematic Reviews* 5:58.

DGAC (Dietary Guidelines Advisory Committee). 2014. *Subcommittee 2: Dietary patterns, foods and nutrients, and health outcomes*. Bethesda, MD: HHS.

Faggion, C. M., Jr. 2015. Critical appraisal of AMSTAR: Challenges, limitations, and potential solutions from the perspective of an assessor. *BMC Medical Research Methodology* 15:63.

Freedman, L. S., A. Schatzkin, D. Midthune, and V. Kipnis. 2011. Dealing with dietary measurement error in nutritional cohort studies. *Journal of the National Cancer Institute* 103(14):1086-1092.

Freedman, L. S., J. M. Commins, W. Willett, L. F. Tinker, D. Spiegelman, D. Rhodes, N. Potischman, M. L. Neuhouser, A. J. Moshfegh, V. Kipnis, D. J. Baer, L. Arab, R. L. Prentice, and A. F. Subar. 2017. Evaluation of the 24-hour recall as a reference instrument for calibrating other self-report instruments in nutritional cohort studies: Evidence from the validation studies pooling project. *American Journal of Epidemiology* 186(1):1-10.

Garner, P., S. Hopewell, J. Chandler, H. MacLehose, E. A. Akl, J. Beyene, S. Chang, R. Churchill, K. Dearness, G. Guyatt, C. Lefebvre, B. Liles, R. Marshall, L. Martínez García, C. Mavergames, M. Nasser, A. Qaseem, M. Sampson, K. Soares-Weiser, Y. Takwoingi, L. Thabane, M. Trivella, P. Tugwell, E. Welsh, E. C. Wilson, and H. J. Schünemann. 2016. When and how to update systematic reviews: Consensus and checklist. *BMJ* 354:i3507.

Goldberg, G. R., A. E. Black, S. A. Jebb, T. J. Cole, P. R. Murgatroyd, W. A. Coward, and A. M. Prentice. 1991. Critical evaluation of energy intake data using fundamental principles of energy physiology: 1. Derivation of cut-off limits to identify under-recording. *European Journal of Clinical Nutrition* 45(12):569-581.

HHS/USDA (U.S. Department of Health and Human Services/U.S. Department of Agriculture). 2013. *The topic formation process*. Bethesda, MD: HHS.

HHS/USDA. 2015a. Dietary Guidelines for Americans *2015 – 2020: Eighth edition*. https://health.gov/dietaryguidelines/2015/guidelines (access July 18, 2017).

HHS/USDA. 2015b. *Scientific report of the 2015 Dietary Guidelines Advisory Committee*. Washington, DC: USDA, Agricultural Research Service.

Higgins, J., and S. Green, editors. 2011. *Cochrane handbook for systematic reviews of interventions, version 5.1.0*, The Cochrane Collaboration.

Hoy, M. K., and J. D. Goldman. 2014. *Calcium intake of the U.S. population: What We Eat in America, NHANES 2009-2010*. Dietary Data Brief No. 13. Beltsville, MD: USDA.

Huang, T. T., S. B. Roberts, N. C. Howarth, and M. A. McCrory. 2005. Effect of screening out implausible energy intake reports on relationships between diet and BMI. *Obesity Research* 13(7):1205-1217.

IOM (Institute of Medicine). 2000. *Dietary Reference Intakes: Applications in dietary assessment.* Washington, DC: National Academy Press.

IOM. 2005. *Dietary Reference Intakes for water, potassium, sodium, chloride, and sulfate.* Washington, DC: The National Academies Press.

IOM. 2011. *Finding what works in health care: Standards for systematic reviews.* Washington, DC: The National Academies Press.

Marcoe, K., W. Juan, S. Yamini, A. Carlson, and P. Britten. 2006. Development of food group composites and nutrient profiles for the MyPyramid food guidance system. *Journal of Nutrition, Education, and Behavior* 38(Suppl 6):S93-S107.

Millen, B. January 10, 2017 (unpublished). *Understanding the committee's methodology for topic formation and reviewing the evidence base.* Presentation to the Committee to Review the Process to Update the *Dietary Guidelines for Americans*, Washington, DC, January 10.

Murphy, S. P., and S. I. Barr. 2006. Recommended dietary allowances should be used to set daily values for nutrition labeling. *American Journal of Clinical Nutrition* 83(5):1223s-1227s.

NCI (National Cancer Institute). 2015. *Usual dietary intakes: The NCI method.* Rockville, MD: NCI.

NCI. 2017. *Dietary assessment primer.* Rockville, MD: NCI.

Prentice, R. L., and Y. Huang. 2011. Measurement error modeling and nutritional epidemiology association analyses. *Canadian Journal of Statistics* 39(3):498-509.

Shea, B., J. Grimshaw, G. Wells, M. Boers, N. Andersson, C. Hamel, A. Porter, P. Tugwell, D. Moher, and L. Bouter. 2007. Development of AMSTAR: A measurement tool to assess the methodological quality of systematic reviews. *BMC Medical Research Methodology* 7(1):10.

Smith, V., D. Devane, C. M. Begley, and M. Clarke. 2011. Methodology in conducting a systematic review of systematic reviews of healthcare interventions. *BMC Medical Research Methodology* 11(1):15.

Tooze, J. A., D. Midthune, K. W. Dodd, L. S. Freedman, S. M. Krebs-Smith, A. F. Subar, P. M. Guenther, R. J. Carroll, and V. Kipnis. 2006. A new statistical method for estimating the usual intake of episodically consumed foods with application to their distribution. *Journal of the American Dietetic Association* 106(10):1575-1587.

Tooze, J. A., V. Kipnis, D. W. Buckman, R. J. Carroll, L. S. Freedman, P. M. Guenther, S. M. Krebs-Smith, A. F. Subar, and K. W. Dodd. 2010. A mixed-effects model approach for estimating the distribution of usual intake of nutrients: The NCI method. *Statistics in Medicine* 29(27):2857-2868.

USDA. 2012. *A series of systematic reviews on the effects of nutrition education on children's and adolescents' dietary intake.* Alexandria, VA: Food and Nutrition Service, USDA.

USDA. 2014. *A series of systematic reviews on the relationship between dietary patterns and health outcomes.* Alexandria, VA: Food and Nutrition Service, USDA.

USDA. 2015. *USDA food patterns.* Washington, DC: USDA.

USDA. 2017. *Nutrition Evidence Library.* Alexandria, VA: Center for Nutrition Policy and Promotion, USDA.

USDA/HHS. 2016 (unpublished). Dietary Guidelines for Americans: *Process brief, sections 4–5.* Prepared for the Committee to Review the Process to Update the Dietary Guidelines for Americans.

USDA/HHS. 2017 (unpublished). Dietary Guidelines for Americans: *Process brief, sections 6–7.* Prepared for the Committee to Review the Process to Update the Dietary Guidelines for Americans.

Viswanathan, M., N. D. Berkman, D. M. Dryden, and L. Hartling. 2012. Development of the RTI item bank on risk of bias and precision of observational studies. *Journal of Clinical Epidemiology* 65(2):163-178.

Viswanathan, M., N. D. Berkman, D. M. Dryden, and L. Hartling. 2013. AHRQ methods for effective health care. In *Assessing risk of bias and confounding in observational studies of interventions or exposures: Further development of the RTI item bank*. Rockville, MD: Agency for Healthcare Research and Quality.

Wegewitz, U., B. Weikert, A. Fishta, A. Jacobs, and D. Pieper. 2016. Resuming the discussion of AMSTAR: What can (should) be made better? *BMC Medical Research Methodology* 16(1):111.

West, S., V. King, T. S. Carey, K. N. Lohr, N. McKoy, S. F. Sutton, and L. Lux. 2002. *Systems to rate the strength of scientific evidence*. Vol. 47. Prepared by the Research Triangle Institute, University of North Carolina Evidence-Based Practice Center. Rockville, MD: Agency for Healthcare Research and Quality.

Whitlock, E. P., J. S. Lin, R. Chou, P. Shekelle, and K. A. Robinson. 2008. Using existing systematic reviews in complex systematic reviews. *Annals of Internal Medicine* 148(10):776-782.

7

Recent Approaches to Assessing Nutritional Adequacy and Exploring Chronic Disease

The recommendations presented in the several editions of the *Dietary Guidelines for Americans* (*DGA*) *Policy Report*[1] have traditionally been oriented toward the healthy U.S. population, ages 2 years and older, and have not been intended for the treatment or management of disease. Over the past several decades the landscape of the general population's health status has shifted. Many Americans now live with one or more chronic disease (Ward et al., 2014). Furthermore, evidence is emerging that exposures to nutrition and other environmental factors in utero and in early life may play a role in "programming" the risk for chronic disease in later life (Hanson and Gluckman, 2015). This places an emphasis on optimizing nutrition and lifestyle in pregnancy and infancy, two population groups previously not included in the *DGA*. The Agricultural Act of 2014 mandated that dietary guidance for these populations be included in the *2020–2025 DGA* (see Chapter 5 for details). Thus, understanding the relationship of diet to chronic disease prevention across the life span and developing relevant guidance in the *DGA* process is important.

This chapter explores how the 2005, 2010, and 2015 Dietary Guidelines Advisory Committees have approached assessing nutritional adequacy[2] and the role of diet in health and chronic disease, noting similarities and

[1] Refer to Chapter 1, Box 1-1, for an explanation of how the term *DGA* is used throughout this National Academies report.

[2] This National Academies committee's Statement of Task used the phrase "nutritional sufficiency." However, to align with standard nomenclature used by the Dietary Reference Intakes, the phrases "nutritional adequacy" and "nutritional inadequacy" will be used in this report.

differences across the different cycles. Opportunities for improvements to the process are also identified.

ASSESSMENTS OF NUTRIENT INTAKE LEVELS OF THE U.S. POPULATION BY THE 2005, 2010, AND 2015 DGACs[3]

The health effects of dietary intake, particularly specific nutrients, are most pronounced at both ends of the spectrum of intake. Deficiencies of an essential nutrient, for example, can lead to nutrient-specific conditions (e.g., iron-deficiency anemia, scurvy, beriberi). Excessive nutrient intake can also lead to adverse effects (e.g., hypercalcemia, hypervitaminosis A). Nutritional adequacy without excessive intake, therefore, is one component for elucidating the relationship between diet and health.

Recent DGACs have evaluated current nutrient intake levels to determine the extent to which the U.S. population is meeting recommended intake goals, primarily as intake relates to the Dietary Reference Intakes (DRIs).[4] The DRIs, defined in Box 7-1, describe nutrient intake requirements averaged over time in apparently healthy individuals. This concept of assessing usual intake is key, as "intake may vary substantially from day to day without ill effect in most cases" (IOM, 2000, p. 3). DRIs serve as benchmarks that can be used to assess inadequacy for a population and for an individual, and also to assess the potential for adverse effects caused by excess. DRIs are set for groups defined by life stage and gender. The framework used to set the current DRIs focuses on intakes that prevent deficiency as well as intakes that prevent adverse effects. Additionally, the existing DRI framework allows for the integration of data on safety, efficacy, and the reduction of chronic diseases, to the extent that specific evidence exists. However, owing to a lack of supporting evidence, few DRI values have been based on chronic disease data (see Appendix E). Efforts are currently under way to move toward using chronic disease end points to establish DRIs.[5]

---

[3] The under- and overconsumption of food groups have also been evaluated by previous DGACs through food pattern modeling and descriptive data analyses. For additional information about such analyses, see Chapter 6.

[4] For additional information about the DRIs, including their evolution and applications, see Appendix E.

[5] A multidisciplinary working group sponsored by the Canadian and U.S. government DRI steering committees met from late 2014 through April 2016 to consider how to base DRI values on chronic disease end points. The working group produced a report that provided extensive discussion of the issues and ideas for paths forward (Yetley et al., 2017). An ad hoc consensus committee of the National Academies of Sciences, Engineering, and Medicine recently released a report in which the options presented by Yetley et al. (2017) are reviewed and recommends methods and guiding principles for including chronic disease end points in the DRI process (NASEM, 2017).

BOX 7-1
Dietary Reference Intakes

Acceptable Macronutrient Distribution Range (AMDR): A range of intakes for a particular energy source that is associated with reduced risk of chronic diseases while providing adequate intakes of essential nutrients (IOM, 2005, p. 14).[a]

Adequate Intake (AI): A recommended average daily nutrient intake level based on observed or experimentally determined approximations or estimates of nutrient intake by a group (or groups) of healthy people that are assumed to be adequate—used when an RDA cannot be determined (IOM, 2003, p. 3).

Estimated Average Requirement (EAR): The average daily nutrient intake level estimated to meet the requirement of half the healthy individuals in a particular life stage and gender group (IOM, 2003, p. 3).

Estimated Energy Requirement (EER): The average dietary energy intake that is predicted to maintain energy balance in a healthy adult of a defined age, gender, weight, height, and level of physical activity consistent with good health. In children and pregnant and lactating women, the EER includes the needs associated with the deposition of tissues or the secretion of milk at rates consistent with good health (IOM, 2005, p. 22).

Recommended Dietary Allowance (RDA): The average daily nutrient intake level sufficient to meet the nutrient requirement of nearly all (97 to 98 percent) healthy individuals in a particular life stage and gender group (IOM, 2003, p. 3).

Tolerable Upper Intake Level (UL): The highest average daily nutrient intake level likely to pose no risk of adverse health effects to almost all individuals in a particular life stage and gender group. As intake increases above the UL, the potential risk of adverse health effects increases (IOM, 2003, p. 3).

[a] This definition changed between the prepublication copy and the final report.

The 2005, 2010, and 2015 DGACs each used the current population intake levels to determine which nutrients are not being consumed at recommended levels. These identified "nutrients of concern" inform the DGACs' food pattern modeling analyses, which ultimately play an integral role in the resulting *DGA* recommendations. The three most recent editions of the *DGA Policy Report*, for instance, have each included guidance on food groups to increase or limit in the diet to address under- and/or overconsumed nutrients (HHS/USDA, 2005a, 2015a; USDA/HHS, 2010a). This guidance ultimately underpins federal nutrition policy, including regulations and nutrition education materials (see Box 1-2 for examples of how the government has applied the *DGA*), and has implications for changes in the food sector. Given this, identification of nutrients of concern appears to be a key step in the overall *DGA* process. The following sections describe how nutrients of concern have been identified and note how the methods and terminology have changed across the three most recent DGACs.

Questions and Data Sources Used to Determine Nutrient Intake Levels of the U.S. Population

In the current process to update the *DGA*, topics and questions reviewed in the scientific report are developed by the DGAC (see Chapter 5 for additional details). The 2005, 2010, and 2015 DGACs each included one or multiple questions related to the current nutrient intake status of the U.S. population. As outlined in Box 7-2, the questions have progressively expanded to include an evaluation of both under- and overconsumption of nutrients and consideration of sources of excesses.

Recent DGACs have relied on national survey data from the What We Eat in America component of the National Health and Nutrition Examination Survey (NHANES)[6] to determine current nutrient intake levels. Both the 2005 and 2010 DGACs used a collection of existing published reports and data tables, which varied in terms of the time span the data reflected, the type of dietary intake represented (i.e., 1-day dietary intake, usual intake), and the analytical approach used. The nutrient intake analyses gathered and performed for the 2015 DGAC, in contrast, used consistent methodologies across a single dataset (2007–2010 NHANES) (HHS/USDA, 2015b).

Classification of Nutrient Intake Levels

Recent DGACs used the analyses of current intakes of the U.S. population to categorize nutrients and identify those that rise to the level "of (public health) concern." Differences exist across the 2005, 2010, and 2015 DGACs with respect to terminology, thresholds used to classify nutrient intake levels, and the extent to which biochemical and health-related data have been incorporated into the process.

[6] The 2005 DGAC used data from the Continuing Survey of Food Intakes by Individuals (CSFII). CSFII was integrated into the National Health and Nutrition Examination Survey (NHANES) in 2002 and is referred to as the "What We Eat in America" component of NHANES (USDA ARS, 2016).

BOX 7-2
Dietary Guidelines Advisory Committee Questions About Nutrient Intake Levels of the U.S. Population

The questions listed below are those posed by the three most recent Dietary Guidelines Advisory Committees to determine nutrients of concern of the U.S. population. Other questions about intake levels of a specific nutrient or of a specific population group have been incorporated in other parts of the scientific reports.

2005 Dietary Guidelines Advisory Committee

- What nutrients are most likely to be consumed by the general public in amounts low enough to be of concern?

2010 Dietary Guidelines Advisory Committee

- What nutrients and dietary components are overconsumed by the general public?
- What nutrients are underconsumed by the general public and present a substantial public health concern?

2015 Dietary Guidelines Advisory Committee

- What are current consumption patterns of nutrients from foods and beverages by the U.S. population?
- Of the nutrients that are underconsumed or overconsumed, including over the Tolerable Upper Limit of Intake (UL), which present a substantial public health concern?
- Is there evidence of overconsumption of any micronutrients from consumption of fortified foods and supplements?

NOTES: The questions listed above are verbatim from the 2005, 2010, and 2015 editions of the *Dietary Guidelines Advisory Committee Scientific Report*. As defined in Box 7-1, the Dietary Reference Intakes refer to the UL as the "Tolerable Upper Intake Level."
SOURCES: HHS/USDA, 2005b, 2015b; USDA/HHS, 2010b.

Terminology Describing Nutrient Intake Levels

As presented in Table 7-1, the terminology used to describe nutrient intake levels has varied across the editions of the *DGAC Scientific Report*. The concept of a "shortfall nutrient" has remained relatively consistent across recent editions of the *DGAC Scientific Report*, describing a nutrient that is underconsumed across the population or in a specific group of the population, relative to DRI values (i.e., Estimated Average Requirement

TABLE 7-1 Terminology Used by the 2005, 2010, and 2015 DGACs to Classify Nutrient Intake Levels

	Descriptions, as Presented in the *DGAC Scientific Report*		
Terminology	2005 DGAC	2010 DGAC	2015 DGAC
Shortfall nutrient	• A nutrient with a high prevalence of inadequate dietary intake • Intake levels are low enough to be of concern	• A high prevalence of inadequate dietary intake among any segment of the population	• A nutrient that is underconsumed across the population or in specific groups relative to the EAR or AI levels
Nutrients that pose special challenges	• Shortfall nutrient for which dietary guidance to meet recommended intake levels was challenging to develop	• N/A	• N/A
Nutrients of concern	• Shortfall nutrients	• Overconsumed nutrients and dietary components • Shortfall nutrients with biochemical indices of nutrient or functional status, when available, and/or disease prevalence data indicating substantial public health significance	• Includes both shortfall nutrients and overconsumed nutrients[a]
Nutrients of public health concern	• N/A	• Synonymous with underconsumed nutrients of concern • Shortfall nutrients, clearly linked to indicators of nutrient inadequacy or disease prevalence and require special consideration in developing dietary guidance to meet recommended food intakes[b]	• Shortfall or overconsumed nutrients with evidence of under- or overconsumption through biochemical nutritional status indicators plus evidence that the nutrient inadequacy or excess is directly related to a specific health condition

TABLE 7-1 Continued

NOTE: AI = Adequate Intake; DGAC = Dietary Guidelines Advisory Committee; EAR = Estimated Average Requirement; N/A = not applicable—phrase not used in the corresponding *DGAC Scientific Report*.

[a] *Nutrients of concern* and *nutrients of public health concern* are defined here as they appear in the introduction of Part D, Chapter 1, of the *2015 DGAC Scientific Report* (HHS/USDA, 2015b). However, later in the chapter, "nutrients of concern" are described as under- and overconsumed nutrients corroborated with biochemical markers of nutritional status, where available, and evidence for associations with health outcomes (HHS/USDA, 2015b).

[b] The 2010 DGAC also used the phrase "nutrients that are underconsumed by the general public and present a substantial public health concern" (USDA/HHS, 2010b).

[EAR] or Adequate Intake [AI]). In the two most recent editions of the *DGAC Scientific Report*, both under- and overconsumed nutrients were included in the classification of "nutrients of (public health) concern." Also emerging in the 2010 and 2015 DGACs was the additional criterion of biochemical indices and/or direct relationship with health conditions as a requisite for a nutrient being classified as being "of (public health) concern." The differentiation between "nutrients of concern" and "nutrients of public health concern," however, has not been consistent across or within the two most recent editions of the *DGAC Scientific Report*.

Intake Level Thresholds Used to Classify Nutrients

The three most recent DGACs all used levels of inadequacy and/or adequacy as the criterion to identify underconsumed nutrients. None, however, explicitly stated a priori criteria or a rationale for the cut-offs used in determining shortfall nutrients. As previously described, the analyses used by the DGACs to assess current intake levels have been heterogeneous. These differences are reflected in the quantitative threshold intake levels of identified shortfall nutrients. Table 7-2 outlines the lowest levels of nutrient inadequacy and the highest levels of nutrient adequacy of the shortfall nutrients identified by the 2005, 2010, and 2015 DGACs.

In addition to assessing underconsumed nutrients, the 2010 and 2015 DGACs also explored overconsumed nutrients. In the *2010 DGAC Scientific Report*, one nutrient was compared to its Tolerable Upper Intake Level (UL) (sodium),[7] while two nutrients with no established ULs (saturated fat and cholesterol) were compared to quantitative intake goals estab-

[7] Select nutrient intakes were compared to the UL in other sections of the 2010 DGAC report, with respect to total dietary intake (i.e., inclusive of dietary supplement intake).

TABLE 7-2 Lowest Levels of Nutrient Inadequacy and Highest Levels of Nutrient Adequacy of Shortfall Nutrients Identified by the 2005, 2010, and 2015 DGACs

Nutrient Characteristic	Threshold Intake Levels of Identified Shortfall Nutrients		
	2005 DGAC	2010 DGAC	2015 DGAC
Nutrients with an EAR	• *Adults:* 58.6 percent or less probability of adequacy • *Children:* 36.5 percent or more of the population with usual intakes below the EAR	• *Adults:* 69 percent or less of the population with intakes above the EAR • *Adolescents:* 71 percent or less of the population with intakes above the EAR[a]	• *Children and Adults:* 37 percent or more of the population below the EAR (U.S. population) • *Adolescents and Premenopausal Women:* 15–16 percent of select population below the EAR for iron • *Children and Adults:* 9 percent of the population below the EAR for folate[b]
Nutrients with an AI	• *Children and Adults:* Mean dietary intakes below the AI	• *Adults:* 36 percent or less of the population with intake above the AI[c] • *Children:* Mean usual intake 76.6 percent or less of the AI[d] • *Children (4–8 years):* 83 percent or less of the population met the AI through all sources[e]	• *Children and Adults:* 5 percent or less of the population with intake above the AI

NOTES: The values presented in this table reflect the lowest level of inadequacy and highest level of adequacy presented as evidence for shortfall nutrients for the population group specified in the corresponding *DGAC Scientific Report*. The values do not reflect a threshold that was explicitly stated as an a priori decision or criterion in the editions of the *DGAC Scientific Report*. AI = Adequate Intake; DGAC = Dietary Guidelines Advisory Committee; EAR = Estimated Average Requirement.

[a] The 2010 DGAC used a U.S. Department of Agriculture Food and Nutrition Service report on intakes of school children as evidence of shortfall nutrients (USDA, 2008). The text indicates the classification was notably due to the intakes of adolescents (USDA/HHS, 2010b). As such, the values in this table reflect the levels of adequacy for children 14 to 18 years of age.

[b] The 2015 DGAC classified folate as an underconsumed nutrient for the U.S. population, ages 2 years and older. Both zinc and vitamin B_6 had higher proportions of the total population with intakes below the EAR than for folate. Levels of intake of folate among adolescents and premenopausal women, however, were at similar levels as those presented in the above table for iron.

TABLE 7-2 Continued

[c] In the *2010 DGAC Scientific Report*, Figures D2.14 and D2.15 provided evidence of which 10 nutrient intakes qualified as tenuous among adult men and women (USDA/HHS, 2010b). Choline was noted as a shortfall nutrient for this population, but it was not included in either figure. As such, the values included in the table only reflect the levels presented in the two figures in the *2010 DGAC Scientific Report*.

[d] The 2010 DGAC used a Food and Nutrition Service report on intakes of school children (USDA, 2008) as evidence of shortfall nutrients. The narrative text indicates the classification of calcium was notably due to the intakes of children 9 to 18 years of age, and the classification of potassium and fiber was based on the intakes of all children (USDA/HHS, 2010b). As such, the values in this table reflect the highest threshold across the noted population age groups.

[e] Based on an analysis by Bailey et al. (2010), which looked at dietary and total usual intakes of calcium and vitamin D. The 2010 DGAC indicated the analysis suggested calcium was a shortfall nutrient for children 4 to 8 years of age.

lished in preceding editions of the *DGA Policy Report* (< 10 percent total energy and < 300 milligrams per day, respectively) (USDA/HHS, 2010b). Although no explicit or a priori cutoff was stated in the *2010 DGAC Scientific Report*, all three nutrients identified as being overconsumed had 50 percent or more of one or multiple population groups exceeding the UL or other standard of excessive intake. In the *2015 DGAC Scientific Report*, an assessment was included of the percentage of the population above the UL for all nutrients evaluated with an established UL. This analysis showed that all but one nutrient (sodium) had 3 percent or less of the population exceeding the UL, suggesting relatively low risk of adverse effects in the general population due to excessive nutrient intake. The 2015 DGAC also used the same intake goals as used by the 2010 DGAC for saturated fat and cholesterol. Again, the assessment was descriptive and no quantitative threshold was explicitly stated for what level of intake in the population or specific group qualified as excessive.

Use of Biochemical and Health-Related Data to Support Classification of Nutrients

As reflected in the terminology used by recent DGACs to classify nutrient intake levels, a progressive shift occurred toward integrating data beyond just nutrient intake levels in the decision-making process for nutrient classification. For example, the primary focus of the 2005 DGAC's assessment of nutrients of concern was on nutrient intake levels. For vitamin E, the 2005 DGAC identified intake levels suggesting widespread deficiency, but this was not accompanied by overt symptoms of deficiency in the U.S. population. Nevertheless, the 2005 DGAC still identified vitamin E as a nutrient of concern based on the dietary intake data alone.

In comparison to the 2005 DGAC's approach, the use of biochemical indicators and other health-related data was more prominent in the 2010 DGAC's categorization of nutrient intakes. Shortfall nutrients were not classified as nutrients of public health concern if a biochemical marker indicated approximately 7 percent or less of the population was inadequate[8] or if the shortfall nutrient did not have nationally representative prevalence data on biochemical or functional deficiency. The 2010 DGAC used data from a variety of sources to justify the selected nutrients of (public health) concern, including biochemical indicator data, evidence presented in a corresponding DRI report supplemented with a literature search of recent publications, an Agency for Healthcare Research and Quality evidence report, and an American Dietetic Association position paper.[9] For some of the nutrients, the evidence was directly linked to a specific question posed by the 2010 DGAC in another section of the scientific report (e.g., "What are the health benefits of dietary fiber?"). For two nutrients the 2010 DGAC identified as being overconsumed (saturated fat and cholesterol), the health-oriented justifications were supported by full Nutrition Evidence Library (NEL) evidence-based reviews conducted to answer specific questions posed by the DGAC elsewhere in the scientific report (i.e., "What is the effect of saturated fat intake on increased risk of cardiovascular disease or type 2 diabetes, including effects on intermediate markers such as serum lipid and lipoprotein levels?" and "What is the effect of dietary cholesterol intake on risk of cardiovascular disease, including effects on intermediate markers such as serum lipid and lipoprotein levels and inflammation?"). The other identified overconsumed nutrient (sodium) was justified by evidence presented in its corresponding DRI report, supplemented with literature published since the DRI report's release.

The 2015 DGAC explicitly stated that it used the totality of evidence from a "three-pronged approach" to determine which under- and overconsumed nutrients posed a substantial public health concern. The three prongs included the dietary intake levels from 2007–2010 NHANES data, analyses from the *Second National Report on Biochemical Indices of Diet and Nutrition in the U.S. Population* (CDC, 2012), and prevalence statistics from the Centers for Disease Control and Prevention. Table 7-3 outlines the extent to which these types of evidence were available and used across the seven identified nutrients of public health concern. Only two of the seven nutrients of public health concern had biochemical indicator data available.

---

[8] This criterion was not explicitly stated by the 2010 DGAC. It was determined by this National Academies committee's review of the evidence presented in the *2010 DGAC Scientific Report*.

[9] The list presented here encompasses all sources used. Some of the listed sources were used for only one of the nutrients.

TABLE 7-3 Evidence Used by the 2015 DGAC to Justify Selection of Nutrients of Public Health Concern

Nutrient	Dietary Intake	Biochemical Indicator[a]	Health Condition	Other Rationale[b]
Calcium	% of population below EAR	No reliable biochemical marker exists	Associated with osteoporosis and other health outcomes	FDA's designation as a nutrient of "public health significance"[c]
Fiber	% of population above the AI[d]	No reliable biochemical marker exists	May play a role in coronary heart disease, colorectal cancer, type 2 diabetes, and obesity	None cited in narrative description
Iron[e]	% of population below EAR	Serum ferritin indicating risk of iron deficiency anemia	Iron-deficiency anemia	FDA's designation as a nutrient of "public health significance"[c]
Potassium	% of population above the AI	Not collected[f]	Associated with hypertension and cardiovascular disease	FDA's designation as a nutrient of "public health significance"[c]
Saturated fat	% of population consuming < 10% of energy from saturated fat[g]	No biochemical indicator data used[h]	Cardiovascular disease	None cited in narrative description
Sodium	% of population above the UL	No biochemical indicator data used[i]	Adverse health events, particularly hypertension	None cited in narrative description
Vitamin D	% of population below EAR	Low serum/plasma 25-hydroxyvitamin D concentrations	High prevalence of osteoporosis and low bone density, particularly in older women	FDA's designation as a nutrient of "public health significance"[c]

NOTE: AI = Adequate Intake; DGAC = Dietary Guidelines Advisory Committee; EAR = Estimated Average Requirement; FDA = U.S. Food and Drug Administration; UL = Tolerable Upper Intake Level.

[a] From the Centers for Disease Control and Prevention's (CDC's) *Second Nutritional Report on Biochemical Indicators of Diet and Nutrition in the U.S. Population* (2012), as part of the 2015 DGAC's "three-pronged approach."

continued

TABLE 7-3 Continued

[b] The information listed in this column was not part of the 2015 DGAC's "three-pronged approach" for classifying nutrients of public health concern, but it was included in the narrative describing the rationale for selecting the nutrients.

[c] Used as evidence by the 2015 DGAC to support its classification.

[d] The AI is based on intake associated with greatest reduction in risk of coronary heart disease.

[e] Only a nutrient of public health concern for adolescent and premenopausal women.

[f] The 2015 DGAC noted that urinary potassium is the primary marker, but it was not collected in the CDC biomarker dataset.

[g] The 2015 DGAC noted that while median intake was not far from the recommended intake of < 10 percent of energy from saturated fat, the majority of the total population exceeded the 10 percent of energy from saturated fat.

[h] No biochemical indicator data from the CDC's *Second Nutritional Report on Biochemical Indicators of Diet and Nutrition in the U.S. Population* (2012) were used to justify the selection of saturated fat as a nutrient of concern. The 2015 DGAC did, however, review existing reports on the relationship between saturated fat and cardiovascular disease in a different chapter of its scientific report (HHS/USDA, 2015b), which included assessing the effects of replacing saturated fatty acids with other types of fatty acids or carbohydrates on low-density lipoprotein (LDL-C), high-density lipoprotein (HDL-C), and triglycerides. The 2015 DGAC broadly pointed to this section of its scientific report to justify the selection of saturated fat as a nutrient of concern, but it did not mention the biochemical markers specifically.

[i] The CDC's *Second Nutritional Report on Biochemical Indicators of Diet and Nutrition in the U.S. Population* (2012) did not include an indicator for sodium. The 2015 DGAC reviewed existing reports on the relationship between sodium and blood pressure in a different chapter of its scientific report (HHS/USDA, 2015b) and broadly pointed to it in its justification of sodium as a nutrient of concern.

Summary of DGAC Assessments of Nutrient Intake Levels of the U.S. Population

This National Academies of Sciences, Engineering, and Medicine (the National Academies) committee's evaluation of the approaches taken to assess and categorize nutrient intake levels of the U.S. population highlights the evolution in the process that has taken place across the three most recent DGACs. The approach has evolved to consider both inadequate and excessive intakes, primarily as dietary intakes relate to the DRIs. The 2015 DGAC was able to apply consistent methodologies to a single dataset across the range of nutrients assessed. The DGACs have progressively shifted to considering evidence beyond just dietary intake data to identify nutrients of (public health) concern. Inconsistences exist in the availability of reliable biochemical data and the use of relationships to health outcomes. Standardization of the process by which nutrients of concern are identified is needed to enhance comparability of analyses across *DGA* cycles and to enhance transparency.

APPROACHES USED BY THE 2005, 2010, AND 2015 DGACs TO EXPLORE HEALTH AND CHRONIC DISEASES

Determining the relationship, effects, and significance of dietary intake on health and risk of chronic disease is more challenging than determining the health effects of inadequate or excessive intake of a single nutrient. Diets are multidimensional and vary by individuals and over time. Dietary intake includes interactions and interdependent relationships across nutrients and other food constituents, adding a layer of complexity to identifying the dietary factor(s) contributing to a given health effect. Chronic diseases are also complex, often exist with multiple morbidities, and develop and progress over long periods of time—even being rooted in exposures during the prenatal period and early infancy (see Chapter 5). The ability to characterize health status is dependent on the existence of a validated biomarker or other measure that represents a discrete state in the causal pathway to chronic disease. It is important to understand how and to what extent diet prevents or contributes to positive or negative health effects, especially in context of other contributing factors. The multifactorial nature of chronic diseases, the complex and dynamic nature of dietary intake, and the strengths and limitations of available evidence ultimately affect what can be explored through the review of the science.

The current DGAC process lacks an analytic framework to structure topic selection, synthesis, and interpretation of the evidence. Recent DGACs have used analytic frameworks to organize individual systematic reviews conducted by the NEL, but such frameworks have not been used to consider the relationships between the questions posed or their purposes. The lack of an analytical framework guiding the overall structure of the evidence review makes it challenging to readily understand the overall approach and to identify gaps. This National Academies committee finds the lack of an analytic framework to be a major limitation of the current process, with respect to understanding the relationship between diet and chronic disease prevention. Recent DGACs have moved toward considering linkages between the specific research questions asked. The 2015 DGAC, for example, identified crosscutting topics that pertained to multiple concepts throughout the scientific report. As will be discussed later in this section, the 2015 DGAC also presented an organizing framework used to structure its scientific report. This framework, however, was largely theoretical.

In the absence of an analytical framework, this National Academies committee reviewed the questions posed by the 2005, 2010, and 2015 DGACs to evaluate what aspects of health and chronic disease status were addressed. The following sections review the DGACs' research questions assessing the relationships between health outcomes and measures and the dietary and nondietary factors considered in questions related to health (e.g., a nutrient, dietary constituent, dietary pattern, behavior, or personal characteristic). Table C-2 in Appendix C provides a summary of the dietary and nondietary factors assessed by each of the three most recent editions of the *DGAC Scientific Report*. For a detailed assessment of the methodological approaches taken to answer the full range of questions posed by the 2015 DGAC, see Chapter 6.

Health Outcomes and Measures of Interest Explicitly Included in Questions

The three most recent editions of the *DGAC Scientific Report* used different types of outcomes and measures in the questions regarding health, which have varied in terms of specificity and scope (see Table C-2). The 2005 DGAC used the term *health* broadly in its research questions, appearing to have used such questions to explore the landscape of the literature and determine which health outcomes or measures have been assessed. The use of general terms was not limited to the 2005 DGAC. The 2010 DGAC measured a number of outcomes of interest, including *health outcomes*, *health effects*, and *health benefits*. However, the 2010 DGAC also narrowed the scope of its research questions by using the phrase *selected health outcomes* to describe a collection of chronic diseases and risk factors including, but not limited to, type 2 diabetes, cardiovascular disease, cancers, and body weight. The 2010 DGAC also posed a range of questions specific to cardiovascular disease and associated risk factors, explicitly naming the health outcome or measure (e.g., inflammation, low-density lipoprotein [LDL] cholesterol levels, coronary heart disease). The 2015 DGAC continued the trend of posing more specific questions. While some questions used broad descriptors (e.g., health benefits, health outcomes, health), many questions explicitly stated the chronic disease or health measure of interest (e.g., breast cancer, cardiovascular disease, obesity). The specificity appears to reflect the guidance provided by the U.S. Department of Agriculture (USDA) and the U.S. Department of Health and Human Services (HHS). During the first meeting of the 2015 DGAC, USDA and HHS suggested that the DGAC explore topics that have the potential to affect food- and nutrition-related health outcomes of public concern, including "body weight status, cardiovascular disease, cancer, as well as type 2 diabetes, bone health, and the prevention of food-borne illness" (HHS/USDA, 2013).

Consideration has also been given to biomarkers and surrogate end points (e.g., LDL cholesterol levels, blood pressure). Although not perfect replacements for clinical end points of chronic disease, validated biomarkers and surrogate end points have a number of strengths that could be leveraged to bolster the evidence base on the relationship between diet and chronic disease. While frameworks for evaluating biomarkers exist, the number of fully validated markers of diet and chronic disease is relatively limited (see Box 4-4 for a discussion of the use of biomarkers to measure dietary intakes) (IOM, 2010, 2016). Furthermore, use of validated biomarkers can lead to misinterpretation of risk if not evaluated in the context of other supporting data (FDA, 2016). Given that the science underlying biomarkers is still emerging, a clear understanding of the proper uses and limitations of such data is necessary for appropriate interpretation and application. Evidence that a systematic process was implemented to evaluate the validity of biomarkers prior to inclusion in a research question or the evidence base by recent DGACs was not immediately available.

The health outcomes of interest were relatively similar across the three most recent editions of the *DGAC Scientific Report*, with each having evaluated the science of dietary intake as it related to cardiovascular disease, cancers, type 2 diabetes, body weight, and blood pressure. DGACs have, however, expanded the set of chronic diseases considered. For example, the 2015 DGAC assessed the effect of dietary patterns on "neurological and psychological illness." Whereas the 2010 DGAC limited its assessments of neurological and psychological illnesses to questions on the relationship between alcohol intake and cognitive decline with age and the effect of maternal intake on infant cognition, the 2015 DGAC placed neurological and psychological illness alongside other widely recognized leading chronic disease (e.g., obesity, cardiovascular disease, type 2 diabetes). The *2015 DGAC Scientific Report* provided the following rationale for inclusion of this health outcome: "[t]he rising numbers of U.S. older adults and the potential human and financial cost of age-related cognitive impairments, such as Alzheimer's disease and other dementias, also have helped drive national interest in chronic mental disease" (HHS/USDA, 2015b). However, no explicit processes or criteria were described for identifying emerging or different health outcomes not included in previous editions of the *DGAC Scientific Report*.

Dietary and Nondietary Factors Included in Questions of Health Outcomes and Measures of Interest

A wide range of dietary and nondietary factors was assessed by the 2005, 2010, and 2015 DGACs in relation to health outcomes and measures of interest. Most of the questions focused on various aspects of dietary intake. All three DGACs, for example, asked questions about the relationship between the intake of a specific nutrient (e.g., sodium, folate, saturated fat) and one or more health outcomes of interest. Although there are similarities across scientific reports with respect to the nutrient-related questions (e.g., the relationship between sodium and blood pressure, health benefits of fiber), many are unique to a single DGAC. Assessments have not been limited to just nutrients. The 2015 DGAC posed questions regarding the relationship between constituents of dietary intake (e.g., caffeine, aspartame, low-calorie sweeteners) and one or more health outcomes or measures. The 2010 DGAC included health outcome–oriented questions about the intake of specific foods (i.e., chocolate, nuts), multivitamin/mineral supplements, and specific sources of nutrients (e.g., plant n-3 fatty acids). The 2010 DGAC also posed questions in which energy appeared to serve as an intermediate link between the dietary intake and health outcome of interest (e.g., "What is the impact of liquids versus solid foods on energy intake and body weight?"). Questions have also assessed broader groupings and descriptors of dietary intake. The 2005 and the 2010 DGACs explored the relationship between intakes of specific food groups (e.g., whole grains, vegetables and fruits) and health outcomes. Other health-oriented questions included measures or descriptors of dietary intake such as energy density, glycemic index and glycemic load, and macronutrient proportions. In a departure from the approaches used in 2005 and 2010, the 2015 DGAC expanded its assessment to include several questions about the relationship between dietary patterns and specific health outcomes.

Not all health-oriented questions posed by recent DGACs focused solely on relationships with measures of dietary intake. Questions exploring factors that have an interconnected relationship with diet and health were included in the 2005, 2010, and 2015 editions of the *DGAC Scientific Report*. The 2005 DGAC, for example, asked questions related to body weight ("How much physical activity is needed to avoid weight regain in weight-reduced persons?"). The 2010 DGAC also asked questions about nondietary factors, such as the relationship between food environment and dietary behaviors on body weight and the relationship between pregnancy weight gain and maternal–child health. By contrast, the 2015 DGAC appears to have been encouraged by USDA and HHS to expand its exploration to topics that have the potential to affect food- and nutrition-related health outcomes of public concern, including "diet-related outcomes relevant to social, behavior[al], environmental topics; intakes of foods; food groups; dietary patterns; nutrients of public health concern; diet quality; and dietary behaviors" (HHS/USDA, 2013). For example, the 2015 DGAC reviewed reports of the relationship between physical activity and a health outcome of interest, as well as the effect of programs, policies, and approaches in various settings (e.g., schools, worksites) on weight status. Other factors explored by the 2015 DGAC included acculturation, household food insecurity, neighborhood and community access to food retail settings, use of diet and body weight self-monitoring strategies, eating out and/or take-away frequency, and frequency and regularity of family shared meals.

Frameworks and Conceptual Models Used by the 2010 and 2015 DGAC and Corresponding Editions of the *DGA Policy Report*

The movement to expand evaluations beyond the effect of dietary intake and health highlights the multifactorial and interconnected nature of diet, health, and a host of other nondietary factors. In its assessment of the low adherence with the *DGA*, the 2010 DGAC pointed to the range of factors that influence food intake and presented a socioecological framework. A modified version of this framework was presented in the *2010 DGA Policy Report*, and was accompanied by a recognition that improvements in health require "comprehensive and coordinated systemwide approaches across [the nation]" (USDA/HHS, 2010a).

Building on the work of the 2010 DGAC, the 2015 DGAC created a conceptual map[10] of the interrelated nature of the influences and outcomes on diet and physical activity patterns and behaviors across the life span (see Figure 7-1). The map was described as providing structure to the

[10] The phrase used by the 2015 DGAC for this visual was "conceptual model." This National Academies committee, however, uses the phrase "conceptual map" instead to be congruous with terminology used throughout this report, which describe models as a computational technique.

2015 DGAC's scientific review of a range of determinants of diet, physical activity behavior, and health and an array of nutrition, physical activity, and related health outcomes. The *2015 DGAC Scientific Report* presented an outline of the factors encompassed by each of the components of the

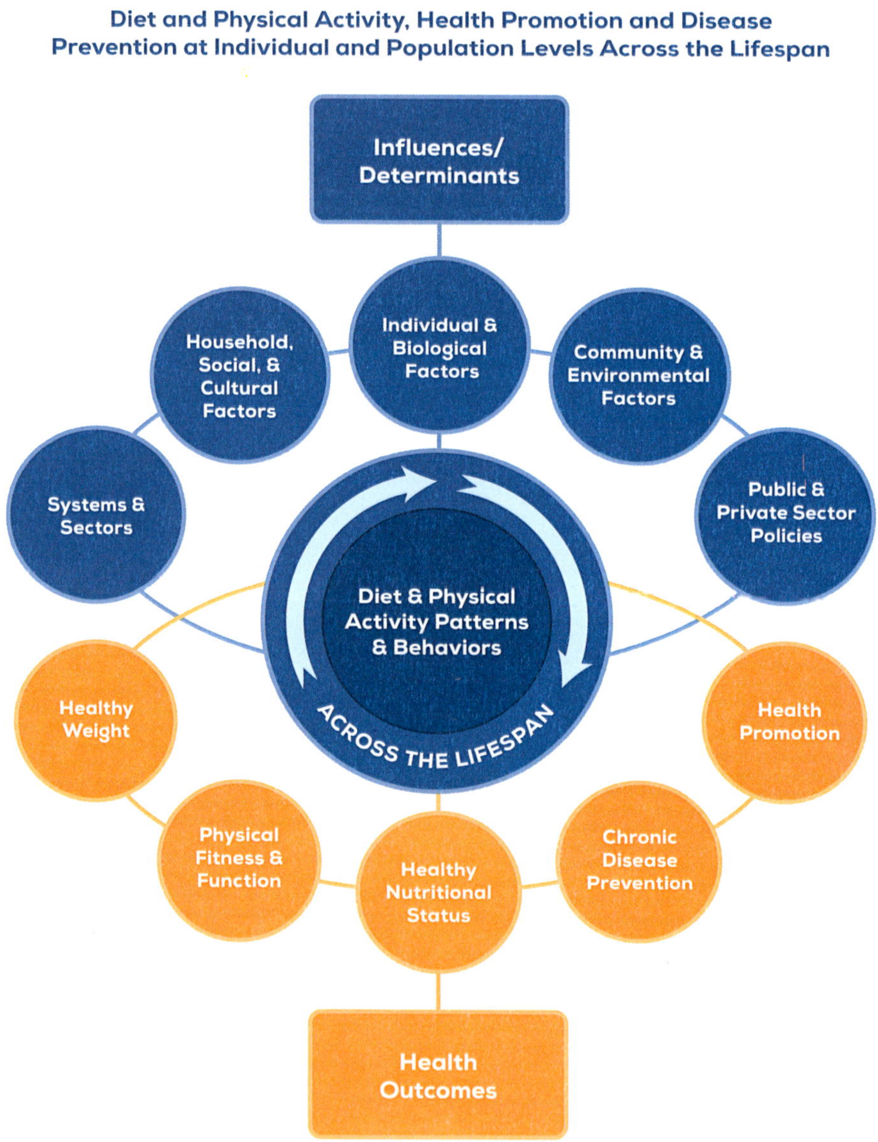

FIGURE 7-1 Conceptual map created by the 2015 DGAC.
SOURCE: Adapted from HHS/USDA, 2015b.

framework and noted which factors were and were not addressed in the DGAC's evidence review. Links, however, were not explicitly drawn between the questions posed by the 2015 DGAC and the conceptual map. The *2015–2020 DGA Policy Report* also presented a social-ecological map for food and physical activity decisions, which differed from the model presented in the *2015 DGAC Scientific Report*. Like its 2010 counterpart, the *2015–2020 DGA Policy Report* map was used to explain and emphasize that multicomponent and multilevel strategies are needed to affect public health.

Summary of DGAC Approaches to Exploring Health and Chronic Diseases

Recent DGACs evaluated a wide range of health-related questions, varying in specificity and in scope. Although the chronic diseases included across the three most recent editions of the *DGAC Scientific Report* have been relatively similar, some expansion of health outcomes has taken place. Recent DGACs were more explicit about the health outcome of interest evaluated and have increasingly assessed the relationship between health and a broader range of nondietary factors. The DGACs' approach to assessing the relationship between diet, health, and chronic disease currently lacks an analytic framework to structure the purpose, function, and relationship of the questions posed. Frameworks presented across the two most recent editions of the *DGAC Scientific Report* and *DGA Policy Report* begin to arrange how the different components and levels interface but remain conceptual in nature.

CONCLUSION

Opportunities exist to improve the process by which the DGAC approaches topics related to dietary intake and health. Using a clear set of terms, establishing one or multiple thresholds for nutrient inadequacy or adequacy that qualifies a nutrient as shortfall, and further integrating biochemical and health-related data in a systematic and consistent manner within and across the editions of the *DGAC Scientific Report* are improvements that may enhance the process by which nutrients of (public health) concern are classified. With respect to chronic disease, opportunities exist to create a process or mechanism by which the DGAC identifies new and emerging health outcomes for review. Related to this concept is the integration of biomarkers and surrogate end point data. While such evidence has the potential to strengthen the dietary recommendations for chronic disease prevention, an examination of the validity and appropriate applications of such data is warranted prior to inclusion into the evidence base. Furthermore, this National Academies committee foresees the creation and use of analytic frameworks to guide topic selection and synthesis and interpretation of evidence as being a valuable addition to the DGAC process. Such an analytic framework would help clarify the purpose of each question, the relationship between questions, what questions are answerable, and what topics need evidence. Finally, this National Academies committee posits that further integrating systems thinking and methods into the *DGA* process would help to better elucidate mechanisms connecting dietary intake and health outcomes.

REFERENCES

Bailey, R. L., K. W. Dodd, J. A. Goldman, J. J. Gahche, J. T. Dwyer, A. J. Moshfegh, C. T. Sempos, and M. F. Picciano. 2010. Estimation of total usual calcium and vitamin D intakes in the United States. *Journal of Nutrition* 140(4):817-822.

CDC (Centers for Disease Control and Prevention). 2012. *Second national report on biochemical indicators of diet and nutrition in the U.S. population.* https://www.cdc.gov/nutritionreport/pdf/nutrition_book_complete508_final.pdf (accessed June 7, 2017).

FDA (U.S. Food and Drug Administration). 2016. *FDA facts: Biomarkers and surrogate endpoints* https://www.fda.gov/aboutfda/innovation/ucm512503.htm (accessed March 16, 2017).

Hanson, M. A., and P. D. Gluckman. 2015. Developmental origins of health and disease—global public health implications. *Best Practice & Research Clinical Obstetrics & Gynaecology* 29(1):24-31.

HHS/USDA (U.S. Department of Health and Human Services/U.S. Department of Agriculture). 2005a. Dietary Guidelines for Americans, *2005*. Washington, DC: U.S. Government Printing Office. https://health.gov/dietaryguidelines/2005.asp (accessed May 31, 2017).

HHS/USDA. 2005b. *The report of the Dietary Guidelines Advisory Committee on* Dietary Guidelines for Americans, *2005*. Washington, DC: Agricultural Research Service, USDA.

HHS/USDA. 2013. *2015 Dietary Guidelines Advisory Committee first meeting transcript.* Bethesda, MD. https://health.gov/dietaryguidelines/2015-BINDER/meeting1/docs/Transcript-Day-2.pdf (accessed May 30, 2017).

HHS/USDA. 2015a. Dietary Guidelines for Americans *2015–2020: Eighth edition.* https://health.gov/dietaryguidelines/2015/guidelines (accessed July 18, 2017).

HHS/USDA. 2015b. *Scientific report of the 2015 Dietary Guidelines Advisory Committee.* Washington, DC: USDA, Agricultural Research Service.

IOM (Institute of Medicine). 2000. *Dietary Reference Intakes: Applications in dietary assessment.* Washington, DC: National Academy Press.

IOM. 2003. *Dietary Reference Intakes: Applications in dietary planning.* Washington, DC: The National Academies Press.

IOM. 2005. *Dietary Reference Intakes for energy, carbohydrate, fiber, fat, fatty acids, cholesterol, protein, and amino acids.* Washington, DC: The National Academies Press.

IOM. 2010. *Evaluation of biomarkers and surrogate endpoints in chronic disease.* Washington, DC: The National Academies Press.

NASEM (National Academies of Sciences, Engineering, and Medicine). 2017. *Guiding principles for developing Dietary Reference Intakes based on chronic disease.* Washington, DC: The National Academies Press.

USDA. 2008. *Diet quality of American school-age children by school lunch participation status: Data from the National Health and Nutrition Examination Survey, 1999-2004.* Alexandria, VA: Food and Nutrition Service.

USDA ARS (Agricultural Research Service). 2016. *What We Eat in America/NHANES overview.* https://www.ars.usda.gov/northeast-area/beltsville-md/beltsville-human-nutrition-research-center/food-surveys-research-group/docs/wweianhanes-overview (accessed July 3, 2017).

USDA/HHS. 2010a. Dietary Guidelines for Americans, *2010. 7th edition*. Washington, DC. https://health.gov/dietaryguidelines/2010 (accessed May 15, 2017).

USDA/HHS. 2010b. *Report of the Dietary Guidelines Advisory Committee on the* Dietary Guidelines for Americans, *2010*. Washington, DC: Agricultural Research Service, USDA.

Ward, B. W., J. S. Schiller, and R. A. Goodman. 2014. Multiple chronic conditions among US adults: A 2012 update. *Preventing Chronic Disease* 11:E62.

Yetley, E. A., A. J. MacFarlane, L. S. Greene-Finestone, C. Garza, J. D. Ard, S. A. Atkinson, D. M. Bier, A. L. Carriquiry, W. R. Harlan, D. Hattis, J. C. King, D. Krewski, D. L. O'Connor, R. L. Prentice, J. V. Rodricks, and G. A. Wells. 2017. Options for basing Dietary Reference Intakes (DRIs) on chronic disease endpoints: Report from a joint US-/Canadian-sponsored working group. *American Journal of Clinical Nutrition* 105(1):249S-285S.

Appendix A

Glossary

conclusion statements—Term used to describe concise statements developed by Dietary Guidelines Advisory Committees (DGACs) to directly answer a specific question.

data integration—In this report, this term refers to the process of combining the results of systematic reviews, food pattern modeling, descriptive data analysis, and any other types of evidence to develop the DGAC's conclusions on the totality of the body of evidence for the *DGA*.

data interpretation—In this report, this term refers to the subjective process of building on synthesis results to develop the DGAC's conclusions about a single study, multiple studies, or systematic reviews (e.g., interpretation of a risk of bias assessment for an individual study; interpretation of heterogeneity across multiple studies to decide whether to combine studies; interpretation of whether or not there is a strong relationship between diet and cardiovascular disease based on a systematic review).

data synthesis—In this report, this term includes both the evaluation of the results across multiple studies in a systematic review (e.g., the qualitative or quantitative analysis of study results), as well as the evaluation of multiple components within a single study (e.g., the combination of correlated outcomes in a single study).

de novo systematic reviews—A type of analysis involving original, comprehensive assessments of the literature.

descriptive data analysis—In this report, this term refers to a type of analysis used by DGACs to answer descriptive questions, generally about overall population trends and population subgroups.

***DGA* cycle**—In this report, this term refers to the 5-year time period between the release of successive editions of the *DGA Policy Report*.

DGA Policy Report—In this report, this term is used to refer to the report released every 5 years by the secretaries of the U.S. Department of Agriculture (USDA) and the U.S. Department of Health and Human Services (HHS) in response to the National Nutrition Monitoring and Related Research Act that is used by policy makers.

***DGA* recommendations**—In this report, this term refers to the main messages from USDA and HHS.

DGAC Scientific Report—In this report, this term is used to describe the technical report that is prepared for the secretaries of USDA and HHS by the DGAC; it serves as the scientific evidence base for developing the *DGA Policy Report*.

evidence grading—The process of determining the strength of a body of evidence in a systematic review, using established criteria.

food pattern modeling—A type of sensitivity analysis used to incorporate various data inputs, constraints, goals, and assumptions to inform food patterns and resulting nutrient profiles, as well as to answer various questions regarding the effects of modifications to food patterns.

guidelines—Term used in the various editions of the *DGA Policy Report* to highlight overarching guidance.

implication statements—Term used by the DGAC to provide context and describe actions that individuals, programs, or policies might take in light of the conclusion statement.

key recommendations—Term used in the various editions of the *DGA Policy Report* to make statements with strong scientific evidence or rationale that will not likely result in substantial changes in the face of new evidence.

nutrient of concern—A nutrient that is under- or overconsumed by the U.S. population and/or select population group, as categorized by the DGAC. The terms *nutrients of concern* and *nutrients of public health concern* were used interchangeably in this report.

Nutrition Evidence Library—A program housed in the USDA's Center for Nutrition Policy and Promotion that conducts systematic reviews to inform federal nutrition policy and programs.

risk of bias assessment—Evaluating the potential for bias in an individual study (e.g., the potential for selection bias in a study).

Appendix B

Public Workshop Agenda and Comments

January 10, 2017
National Academy of Sciences Building—Lecture Room
2101 Constitution Avenue, NW
Washington, DC 20418

8:30 **Welcome and Introductory Remarks**
Rob Russell, Chair

8:35 **Lessons from the 2015 Dietary Guidelines Advisory Committee (DGAC)**
- Barbara Millen, former chair, 2015 DGAC

9:20 **Systematic Reviews in Nutrition**
- Stephanie Chang, Agency for Healthcare Research and Quality
- Eve Essery Stoody, U.S. Department of Agriculture (USDA)
- Julie Obbagy, USDA

10:40 **Developing and Planning for Systematic Reviews**
- Shawna Mercer, Centers for Disease Control and Prevention
- Holger Schünemann, McMaster University (remote)
- David Meltzer, University of Chicago (remote)

1:15 **The Role of Nutrition and Diet in Preventing and Treating Chronic Disease**
- Bert Garza, Boston College and Johns Hopkins University

1:45 **Other Data Inputs into the *DGA***
- Patricia Britten, former USDA
- Patricia Mabry, Indiana University

3:00 Dissemination and Implementation of the *DGA*

- Kathleen Rasmussen, Cornell University
- Janet de Jesus, National Institutes of Health
- Becky Domokos-Bays, Supervisor of School Nutrition, Loudoun County

At the workshop, the committee asked for a public response to two questions:

- What are the two major challenges you face in implementing the *DGA*?
- What are the two biggest opportunities you see for the *DGA* to promote chronic disease prevention and ensure nutritional sufficiency?

Responses from the public were made in person during the workshop and received online from the following individuals and groups:

Angela Amico, Center for Science in the Public Interest, on behalf of Lorrene Ritchie, University of California Nutrition Policy Institute
Tejas Bhatt, Institute of Food Technologists
Darlena Birch, National Women, Infants, and Children Association
Cara Brumfield, 1,000 Days
Robert Burns, Grocery Manufacturers Association
Jeannette Crenshaw, United States Breastfeeding Committee
Emma Gregory, American Frozen Food Institute
Colette Heimowitz, Atkins Nutritionals, Inc.
Guy Johnson, McCormick Science Institute
Casey Keller, Global Wrigley
Mark Kennedy, Physicians Committee for Responsible Medicine
Clara Lau, National Cattlemen's Beef Association
Susan Levin, Physicians Committee for Responsible Medicine
Sean Lucan, Albert Einstein College of Medicine
Richard Lucas, Food and Nutrition Service, U.S. Department of Agriculture
Jim O'Hara, Center for Science in the Public Interest
Sarah Ohlhorst, American Society for Nutrition
Mary Pat Raimondi, Academy of Nutrition and Dietetics
Tia Rains, Egg Nutrition Center
Pauline Sakamoto, Human Milk Banking Association of North America
Lee Sanders, American Bakers Association
Kristen Strader, Public Citizen
Paula Trumbo, U.S. Food and Drug Administration
Joan Younger, American Academy of Pediatrics Section on Breastfeeding
Tracey Ziener, Wrigley

Appendix C

DGAC Topics and Questions

This appendix contains two parts. The first part lists the questions addressed in the *2015 DGAC Scientific Report*, arranged by the source of evidence as recorded in that report (HHS/USDA, 2015). Questions that were addressed with more than one source of evidence are listed under the source occurring first in this list and clarified in footnotes. The second part is Table C-1, which lists the dietary and nondietary factors assessed in relation to health status and chronic disease explicitly stated in the questions addressed in the 2005, 2010, and 2015 editions of the *DGAC Scientific Report*.

QUESTIONS ADDRESSED IN THE *2015 DGAC SCIENTIFIC REPORT*

Systematic Reviews
(de novo Nutrition Evidence Library [NEL] Systematic Review)

- What is the relationship between dietary patterns and risk of cancer?
- What is the relationship between dietary patterns and risk of congenital anomalies?
- What is the relationship between dietary patterns and risk of neurological and psychological illnesses?
- What is the relationship between dietary patterns and bone health?
- What is the relationship between eating out and/or take away meals and body weight in children and adults?

- What is the relationship between frequency and regularity of family shared meals and measures of dietary intake in U.S. population groups?
- What is the relationship between frequency and regularity of family shared meals and measures of body weight and obesity in U.S. population groups?
- What is the relationship between sedentary behavior and measures of dietary intake and body weight in adults?
- What is the relationship between use of diet and body weight self-monitoring strategies and body weight outcomes in adults and youth?
- What is the relationship between knowledge and use of food and menu labels and measures of dietary intake in U.S. population groups?
- What is the relationship between household food insecurity (HFI) and measures of dietary intake and body weight?
- What is the relationship between acculturation and measures of dietary intake?
- What is the relationship between acculturation and body weight?
- What is the relationship between acculturation and risk of cardiovascular disease (CVD)?
- What is the relationship between acculturation and risk of type 2 diabetes?
- What is the relationship between neighborhood and community access to food retail settings and individuals' dietary intake and quality?
- What is the relationship between neighborhood and community access to food retail settings and weight status?
- What is the impact of obesity prevention approaches in early care and education programs on the weight status of children ages 2 to 5 years?[1]
- What is the relationship between population-level dietary patterns and long-term food sustainability?
- What consumer behaviors prevent food safety problems?[2]
- What is the relationship between sodium intake and blood pressure in children?[3]
- What is the relationship between sodium intake and cardiovascular disease outcomes?[3]

---

[1] Existing systematic review used in addition to the NEL systematic review.
[2] Topic update from the 2010 DGAC report; no new systematic review conducted.
[3] Update of the 2010 NEL systematic review.

- What is the relationship between the intake of added sugars and cardiovascular disease, body weight/obesity, type 2 diabetes, and dental caries?[4]

Existing Systematic Reviews and Reports

- What is the relationship between dietary patterns and risk of cardiovascular disease?
- What is the relationship between dietary patterns and measures of body weight or obesity?
- What is the relationship between dietary patterns and risk of type 2 diabetes?
- How effective are behavioral interventions in youth that focus on reducing recreational sedentary screen time and improving physical activity and/or diet?
- What is the impact of school-based approaches on the dietary intake, quality, behaviors, and/or preference of school-aged children?
- What is the impact of school-based policies on the dietary intake, quality, behaviors, and/or preferences of school-aged children?
- What is the impact of school-based approaches on the weight status of school-aged children?
- What is the impact of school-based policies on the weight status of school-aged children?
- What is the impact of worksite-based approaches on the dietary intake, quality, behaviors, and/or preferences of employees?
- What is the impact of worksite policies on the dietary intake, quality, behaviors, and/or preferences of employees?
- What is the impact of worksite-based approaches on the weight status of employees?
- What is the impact of worksite policies on the weight status of employees?
- What are the comparative nutrient profiles of current farm-raised versus wild caught seafood?
- What are the comparative contaminant levels of current farm-raised versus wild caught seafood?[5]
- What is the worldwide capacity to produce farm-raised versus wild-caught seafood that is nutritious and safe for Americans?

---

[4] Cardiovascular disease addressed with an NEL systematic review; body weight/obesity, type 2 diabetes, and dental caries addressed with existing reports.

[5] Data analysis used in addition to existing systematic reviews.

- What is the relationship between usual coffee/caffeine consumption and health?
- What is the relationship between high-dose caffeine consumption and health?
- What is the relationship between aspartame consumption and health?
- What is the relationship between sodium intake and blood pressure in adults?
- What effect does the interrelationship of sodium and potassium have on blood pressure and cardiovascular disease outcomes?
- What is the relationship between intake of saturated fat and risk of cardiovascular disease?
- What is the relationship between the intake of low-calorie sweeteners and body weight/obesity and type 2 diabetes?
- What is the relationship between physical activity, body weight, and health outcomes in children and adolescents?
- What is the relationship between physical activity and body weight?
- What is the relationship between physical activity and cardiorespiratory health?
- What is the relationship between physical activity and metabolic health and risk of type 2 diabetes?
- What is the relationship between physical activity and musculoskeletal health?
- What is the relationship between physical activity and incidence of breast and colon cancer?
- What is the relationship between physical activity and mental health?
- What is the relationship between physical activity and health outcomes in people with disabilities?
- Does being physically active during pregnancy and the postpartum period provide health benefits?
- What is the relationship between the amount and type of physical activity and the risk of adverse events?
- What dose of physical activity is most likely to provide health benefits in children and adolescents?
- What dose of physical activity is most likely to provide health benefits in adults?
- Are there any special considerations for dose of physical activity for older adults?
- What is the relationship between physical activity participation and interventions in school-based settings?

- What is the relationship between physical activity participation and interventions to change the built environment?
- What is the relationship between physical activity participation and interventions based in home settings?
- What is the relationship between physical activity participation and interventions based in early care and education centers?
- What is the relationship between physical activity participation and interventions based in primary health care settings?

Food Pattern Modeling

- How well do updated U.S. Department of Agriculture (USDA) Food Patterns meet Institute of Medicine (IOM) Dietary Reference Intakes and 2010 *Dietary Guidelines* recommendations? How do the recommended amounts of food groups compare to current distributions of usual intakes for the U.S. population?
- How well do the USDA Food Patterns meet the nutritional needs of children 2 to 5 years of age, and how do the recommended amounts compare to their current intakes? Given the relatively small empty calorie limit for this age group, how much flexibility is possible in food choices?
- Can vitamin D Estimated Average Requirements and/or Recommended Dietary Allowances be met with careful food choices following recommended amounts from each food group in the USDA Food Patterns? How restricted would food choices be, and how much of the vitamin D would need to come from fortified dairy and other food products?
- Using the food pattern modeling process, can healthy eating patterns for vegetarians and for those who want to follow a Mediterranean-style diet be developed? How do these patterns differ from the USDA Food Patterns previously updated for use by the 2015 DGAC?

Descriptive Data Analyses

- What are current consumption patterns of nutrients from foods and beverages by the U.S. population?
- Of the nutrients that are underconsumed or overconsumed, including over the Tolerable Upper Limit of Intake (UL), which present a substantial public health concern?
- What would be the effect on food choices and overall nutrient adequacy of limiting saturated fatty acids to 6 percent of total calories by substituting mono- and polyunsaturated fatty acids?

- Is there evidence of overconsumption of any micronutrients from consumption of fortified foods and supplements?
- What is the level of caffeine intake derived from foods and beverages on the basis of IOM Dietary Reference Intakes age and sex categories in the U.S. population?
- What are current consumption patterns of USDA Food Pattern food groups by the U.S. population?
- What is the contribution of whole grain foods, fruits and vegetables, and other food groups to (1) total fiber intake and (2) total nutrient intake in the USDA Food Patterns? What is the contribution of fruit and vegetables to current nutrient intake (focus on nutrients of concern, including fiber)?
- What would be the impact on the adequacy of the patterns if (1) no dairy foods were consumed, (2) if calcium was obtained from nondairy sources (including fortified foods), and (3) if the proportions of milk and yogurt to cheese were modified? What is the relationship between changes in types of beverages consumed (milk compared with sugar-sweetened beverages) and diet quality?
- What are the trends in USDA Food Pattern food group consumption by the U.S. population?
- What are the current consumption patterns by food categories (i.e., foods as consumed) by the U.S. population?
- What are the top foods contributing to energy intake by the U.S. population?
- What are the top foods contributing to sodium, saturated fat, and added sugars intake by the U.S. population?
- What is the current contribution of fruit products with added sugars to intake of added sugars?
- What is the current contribution of vegetable products with added sodium to intake of sodium?
- What is the current contribution of refined grains to intake of added sugars, saturated fat, some forms of polyunsaturated fat, and sodium?
- What are the sources of caffeine from foods and beverages on the basis of age and sex subgroups?
- What is the contribution of beverage types to energy intake by the U.S. population?
- What are the current status and trends in the number of daily eating occasions and frequency of meal skipping? How do diet quality and energy content vary based on eating occasion?

- What are the current status and trends in the location of meal and snack consumption and sources of food and beverages consumed at home and away from home? How do diet quality and energy content vary based on the food and beverage source?
- What is the current prevalence of overweight/obesity and distribution of body weight, body mass index (BMI), and abdominal obesity in the U.S. population and in specific age, sex, race/ethnicity and income groups? What are the trends in prevalence?
- What is the relative prevalence of metabolic and cardiovascular risk factors (i.e., blood pressure, blood lipids, and diabetes) by BMI/waist circumference in the U.S. population and specific population groups?
- What are the current rates of nutrition-related health outcomes (i.e., incidence of and mortality from cancer [breast, lung, colorectal, and prostate] and prevalence of cardiovascular disease, high blood pressure, diabetes, bone health, congenital anomalies, and neurological and psychological illness) in the overall U.S. population?
- What is the composition of dietary patterns with evidence of positive health outcomes (e.g., Mediterranean-style patterns, Dietary Approaches to Stop Hypertension [DASH]-style patterns, patterns that closely align with the Healthy Eating Index, and vegetarian patterns) and of patterns commonly consumed in the United States? What are the similarities (and differences) within and among the dietary patterns with evidence of positive health outcomes and the commonly consumed dietary patterns?
- To what extent does the U.S. population consume a dietary pattern that is similar to those observed to have positive health benefits (e.g., Mediterranean-style patterns, Dietary Approaches to Stop Hypertension [DASH]-style patterns, patterns that closely align with the Healthy Eating Index, and vegetarian patterns) overall and by age/sex and race/ethnic groups?

REFERENCES

HHS/USDA (U.S. Department of Health and Human Services/U.S. Department of Agriculture). 2005. *The report of the Dietary Guidelines Advisory Committee on* Dietary Guidelines for Americans, *2005*. Washington, DC: Agricultural Research Service, USDA.

HHS/USDA. 2015. *Scientific report of the 2015 Dietary Guidelines Advisory Committee.* Washington, DC: USDA, Agricultural Research Service.

USDA/HHS. 2010. *Report of the Dietary Guidelines Advisory Committee on the* Dietary Guidelines for Americans, *2010*. Washington, DC: Agricultural Research Service, USDA.

TABLE C-1 Similarities and Differences of the Dietary and Nondietary Factors Assessed in Relation to Health Status and Chronic Disease Explicitly Included in Questions Addressed in the 2005, 2010, and 2015 Editions of the *DGAC Scientific Report*

Health Outcomes and Measures Used in DGAC Question	Dietary and Nondietary Factors Assessed with Respect to Health Status or Chronic Disease		
	2005 DGAC	2010 DGAC	2015 DGAC
General			
Adverse health effects	• N/A	• Alcohol consumption during lactation	• N/A
Health	• Recommended amount of fluids • Relationship with intake fats[c] and with select food groups[d] • Effect of salt (sodium chloride) intake and potassium intake • Importance of glycemic response to carbohydrates • Significance of added sugars intake	• Role of prebiotics and probiotics	• Relationship with select dietary components[e] and with physical activity and body weight
Health benefits	• Of fiber-containing foods	• Of dietary fiber	• Physical activity[a] • Dose of physical activity
Health effects	• N/A	• Consumption of nuts and of chocolate	• N/A
Health outcomes	• N/A	• Comparison of a vegetarian diet versus a diet that customarily includes animal products • Relationship with physical activity and body weight	• Relationship with physical activity[b]

Maternal–child health	• N/A	• Relationship with maternal weight gain	• N/A
Other nutrition-related aspects of health	• Relationship with physical activity	• N/A	• N/A
Prevent chronic disease	• N/A	• Multivitamin/mineral supplement	• N/A
Risk of adverse events	• N/A	• N/A	• Relationship with physical activity[f]
Selected health outcomes	• N/A	• Relationship with select food groups[g] and with glycemic index and glycemic load • Effect of weight loss versus weight maintenance and of maternal dietary intake of seafood n-3 fatty acids[h]	• N/A
Several major causes of death (cardiovascular disease, cancer, and trauma)	• Dose–response relationship with alcohol intake	• N/A	• N/A
Related to Body Weight			
Abdominal obesity	• N/A	• N/A	• Prevalence, trends
Body mass index	• Relationship with consumption of energy-dense food	• N/A	• Prevalence, trends

continued

TABLE C-1 Continued

Health Outcomes and Measures Used in DGAC Question	Dietary and Nondietary Factors Assessed with Respect to Health Status or Chronic Disease		
	2005 DGAC	2010 DGAC	2015 DGAC
Body weight	• Relationship with physical activity	• Relationship with select measures of dietary intake[i] and with physical activity and other outcomes • Effects of the food environment and dietary behaviors and of liquid versus solid foods	• Prevalence, trends • Relationship with dietary patterns, with factors related to meals,[j] with sedentary behavior, with select demographic characteristics,[k] with intake of select dietary components,[l] with physical activity behaviors,[m] and with diet and body weight self-monitoring strategies
Childhood adiposity	• N/A	• Relationship with dietary intake	• N/A
Obesity	• N/A	• N/A	• Relationship with dietary patterns, with frequency, regularity of family shared meals, and with select dietary components[n]
Overweight/obesity	• N/A	• N/A	• Prevalence, trends
Weight gain	• N/A	• Relationship with alcohol intake	• N/A
Weight loss	• Optimal proportions of dietary fat and carbohydrates	• Relationship with dietary energy density	• N/A
Weight maintenance	• Optimal proportions of dietary fat and carbohydrates	• N/A	• N/A

Weight status	• N/A	• N/A	• Relationship with neighborhood and community access to food retail settings • Effect of policies and approaches[o]
Related to Cardiovascular Status			
Cardiorespiratory health	• N/A	• N/A	• Relationship with physical activity
Cardiovascular disease	• Relationship with cholesterol intake	• Relationship with seafood and with plant n-3 fatty acids • Effect of intake of fats[p]	• Prevalence • Relationship with dietary patterns, with acculturation, and with intakes of select nutrients[q]
Coronary heart disease	• N/A	• Relationship with alcohol intake	• N/A
(High) blood pressure	• N/A	• Effect of sodium intake	• Prevalence • Relationship with select nutrients[r]
Inflammation	• N/A	• Effect of n-6 polyunsaturated fatty acid intake	• N/A
LDL cholesterol	• N/A	• Effect of dietary stearic acid	• N/A
LDL-, HDL- and non-HDL cholesterol levels	• N/A	• Effect of consuming natural versus synthetic *trans* fatty acids	• N/A
Metabolic and cardiovascular risk factors (i.e., blood pressure, blood lipids, and diabetes)	• N/A	• N/A	• Relative prevalence

continued

TABLE C-1 Continued

Health Outcomes and Measures Used in DGAC Question	Dietary and Nondietary Factors Assessed with Respect to Health Status or Chronic Disease		
	2005 DGAC	2010 DGAC	2015 DGAC
Serum lipid and lipoprotein levels	• N/A	• Effect of select fats[s]	• N/A
Related to Cancer			
Cancer	• N/A	• N/A	• Relationship with dietary patterns
Breast cancer	• N/A	• N/A	• Incidence, mortality rates • Relationship with physical activity[t]
Colorectal cancer	• N/A	• N/A	• Incidence, mortality rates • Relationship with physical activity[u]
Lung cancer	• N/A	• N/A	• Incidence, mortality rates
Prostate cancer	• N/A	• N/A	• Incidence, mortality rates
Related to Diabetes and Metabolic Health			
(Type 2) diabetes	• N/A	• Effect of select fats[v]	• Prevalence • Relationship with dietary patterns, with acculturation, with select dietary components,[w] and physical activity and metabolic health
Metabolic health	• N/A	• N/A	• Relationship with physical activity and type 2 diabetes

Related to Mental Health			
Cognitive decline with age	• N/A	• Relationship with alcohol intake	• N/A
Mental health	• N/A	• N/A	• Relationship with physical activity
Neurological and psychological illness	• N/A	• N/A	• Prevalence • Relationship with dietary patterns
Other			
Bone health	• N/A	• Relationship with alcohol intake	• Prevalence • Relationship with dietary patterns
Congenital anomalies	• N/A	• N/A	• Prevalence • Relationship with dietary patterns
Dental caries	• Relationship with carbohydrate intake	• N/A	• Relationship with added sugars intake
Musculoskeletal health	• N/A	• N/A	• Relationship with physical activity
Total mortality	• Dose-response relationship with alcohol intake	• N/A	• N/A

NOTE: DGAC = Dietary Guidelines Advisory Committee; N/A = not applicable—phrase not used in the corresponding *DGAC Scientific Report*.

[a] During pregnancy and postpartum period.

[b] The question was specific to people with disabilities.

[c] Includes separate questions for the relationship between health and intake of total fat, *trans* fat, n-6 polyunsaturated fatty acids, n-3 fatty acids, and monounsaturated fatty acids.

[d] Includes separate questions for the relationship between health and intake of fruit and vegetable, whole grains, and milk products.

[e] Includes separate questions for the relationship between health and usual coffee/caffeine consumption, high-dose caffeine consumption, and aspartame consumption.

[f] Amount and type.

continued

TABLE C-1 Continued

[g] Includes separate questions for the relationship between health and intake of animal protein products, vegetable and/or soy protein, milk and milk products, cooked dry beans and peas, whole grains, and vegetables and whole fruit intake, excluding juice.

[h] Effect on breastmilk composition and health outcomes in infants.

[i] Includes separate questions about the relationship between body weight and macronutrient proportion, sugar-sweetened beverage intake and energy intake, and non-caloric sweeteners and energy intake.

[j] Includes separate questions about the relationship between body weight and eating out and/or take away meals, and the frequency and regularity of family shared meals.

[k] Includes separate questions about the relationship between body weight and acculturation and household food insecurity.

[l] Includes separate questions about the relationship between body weight and intake of low-calorie sweeteners and intake of added sugars.

[m] Includes separate questions about the relationship between body weight and sedentary behaviors, physical activity, and physical activity and health.

[n] Includes separate questions about low-calorie sweeteners and added sugars intake.

[o] Includes separate questions on the effect of obesity prevention approaches in early care and education programs, school-based approaches, school-based policies, worksite-based approaches, and worksite policies.

[p] Includes separate questions on the risk of cardiovascular disease and intake of saturated fat, cholesterol, monounsaturated fatty acids (when substituted for saturated fatty acids), and n-6 polyunsaturated fatty acids.

[q] Includes separate questions on the relationship between cardiovascular disease and intake of sodium, added sugars, saturated fat, and the interrelationship of sodium and potassium.

[r] Includes separate questions on the relationship between blood pressure and intake of sodium and the interrelationship of sodium and potassium.

[s] Includes separate questions about the effects of saturated fat intake, monounsaturated fatty acid intake (when substituted for saturated fatty acids), and n-6 polyunsaturated fatty acid intake on risk of type 2 diabetes.

[t] Relationship explored was with breast cancer incidence.

[u] Relationship explored was with colon cancer incidence.

[v] Includes separate questions about the effects of saturated fat intake, monounsaturated fatty acid intake (when substituted for saturated fatty acids), and n-6 polyunsaturated fatty acid intake on risk of type 2 diabetes. Also, the effect of replacing a high carbohydrate diet with a high monounsaturated fatty acid diet in persons with type 2 diabetes.

[w] Includes separate questions about the relationship between type 2 diabetes and intake of low-calorie sweeteners and intake of added sugars.

SOURCES: HHS/USDA, 2005, 2015; USDA/HHS, 2010.

Appendix D

Dietary Guidelines for Americans Guidelines and Key Recommendations

1980 *DIETARY GUIDELINES FOR AMERICANS*

The 1980 *Dietary Guidelines for Americans* presented seven guidelines (USDA/HHS, 1980):

- Eat a variety of foods.
- Maintain ideal weight.
- Avoid too much fat, saturated fat, and cholesterol.
- Eat foods with adequate starch and fiber.
- Avoid too much sugar.
- Avoid too much sodium.
- If you drink alcohol, do so in moderation.

1985 *DIETARY GUIDELINES FOR AMERICANS*

The 1985 *Dietary Guidelines for Americans* presented seven guidelines (USDA/HHS, 1985):

- Eat a variety of foods.
- Maintain desirable weight.
- Avoid too much fat, saturated fat, and cholesterol.
- Eat foods with adequate starch and fiber.
- Avoid too much sugar.
- Avoid too much sodium.
- If you drink alcoholic beverages, do so in moderation.

1990 *DIETARY GUIDELINES FOR AMERICANS*

The 1990 *Dietary Guidelines for Americans* presented seven guidelines (USDA/HHS, 1990):

- Eat a variety of foods.
- Maintain healthy weight.
- Choose a diet low in fat, saturated fat, and cholesterol.
- Choose a diet with plenty of vegetables, fruits, and grain products.
- Use sugars only in moderation.
- Use salt and sodium only in moderation.
- If you drink alcoholic beverages, do so in moderation.

1995 *DIETARY GUIDELINES FOR AMERICANS*

The 1995 *Dietary Guidelines for Americans* presented seven guidelines (USDA/HHS, 1995):

- Eat a variety of foods.
- Balance the food you eat with physical activity—maintain or improve your weight.
- Choose a diet with plenty of grain products, vegetables, and fruits.
- Choose a diet low in fat, saturated fat, and cholesterol.
- Choose a diet moderate in sugars.
- Choose a diet moderate in salt and sodium.
- If you drink alcoholic beverages, do so in moderation.

2000 *DIETARY GUIDELINES FOR AMERICANS*

The 2000 *Dietary Guidelines for Americans* contained 10 guidelines clustered into 3 messages (USDA/HHS, 2000):

10 Guidelines

- Aim for a healthy weight.
- Be physically active each day.
- Let the Pyramid guide your food choices.
- Choose a variety of grains daily, especially whole grains.
- Choose a variety of fruits and vegetables daily.
- Keep food safe to eat.
- Choose a diet that is low in saturated fat and cholesterol and moderate in total fat.
- Choose beverages and foods to moderate your intake of sugars.

- Choose and prepare foods with less salt.
- If you drink alcoholic beverages, do so in moderation.

3 Messages

- Aim for fitness.
- Build a healthy base.
- Choose sensibly.

2005 *DIETARY GUIDELINES FOR AMERICANS*

The 2005 *Dietary Guidelines for Americans* had 41 key recommendations, 23 of which were for the general population and 18 for specific population groups (HHS/USDA, 2005).

Adequate Nutrients Within Calorie Needs

Key Recommendations

- Consume a variety of nutrient-dense foods and beverages within and among the basic food groups while choosing foods that limit the intake of saturated and *trans* fats, cholesterol, added sugars, salt, and alcohol.
- Meet recommended intakes within energy needs by adopting a balanced eating pattern, such as the U.S. Department of Agriculture (USDA) Food Guide or the Dietary Approaches to Stop Hypertension (DASH) Eating Plan.

Key Recommendations for Specific Population Groups

- *People over age 50.* Consume vitamin B_{12} in its crystalline form (i.e., fortified foods or supplements).
- *Women of childbearing age who may become pregnant.* Eat foods high in heme iron and/or consume iron-rich plant foods or iron-fortified foods with an enhancer of iron absorption, such as vitamin C–rich foods.
- *Women of childbearing age who may become pregnant and those in the first trimester of pregnancy.* Consume adequate synthetic folic acid daily (from fortified foods or supplements) in addition to food forms of folate from a varied diet.
- *Older adults, people with dark skin, and people exposed to insufficient ultraviolet band radiation (i.e., sunlight).* Consume extra vitamin D from vitamin D–fortified foods and/or supplements.

Weight Management

Key Recommendations

- To maintain body weight in a healthy range, balance calories from foods and beverages with calories expended.
- To prevent gradual weight gain over time, make small decreases in food and beverage calories and increase physical activity.

Key Recommendations for Specific Population Groups

- *Those who need to lose weight.* Aim for a slow, steady weight loss by decreasing calorie intake while maintaining an adequate nutrient intake and increasing physical activity.
- *Overweight children.* Reduce the rate of body weight gain while allowing growth and development. Consult a health care provider before placing a child on a weight-reduction diet.
- *Pregnant women.* Ensure appropriate weight gain as specified by a health care provider.
- *Breastfeeding women.* Moderate weight reduction is safe and does not compromise weight gain of the nursing infant.
- *Overweight adults and overweight children with chronic diseases and/or on medication.* Consult a health care provider about weight loss strategies prior to starting a weight-reduction program to ensure appropriate management of other health conditions.

Physical Activity

Key Recommendations

- Engage in regular physical activity and reduce sedentary activities to promote health, psychological well-being, and a healthy body weight.
    - To reduce the risk of chronic disease in adulthood: Engage in at least 30 minutes of moderate-intensity physical activity, above usual activity, at work or home on most days of the week.
    - For most people, greater health benefits can be obtained by engaging in physical activity of more vigorous intensity or longer duration.
    - To help manage body weight and prevent gradual, unhealthy body weight gain in adulthood: Engage in approximately 60 minutes of moderate- to vigorous-intensity activity on

most days of the week while not exceeding caloric intake requirements.
   - To sustain weight loss in adulthood: Participate in at least 60 to 90 minutes of daily moderate-intensity physical activity while not exceeding caloric intake requirements. Some people may need to consult with a health care provider before participating in this level of activity.
- Achieve physical fitness by including cardiovascular conditioning, stretching exercises for flexibility, and resistance exercises or calisthenics for muscle strength and endurance.

Key Recommendations for Specific Population Groups

- *Children and adolescents.* Engage in at least 60 minutes of physical activity on most, preferably all, days of the week.
- *Pregnant women.* In the absence of medical or obstetric complications, incorporate 30 minutes or more of moderate-intensity physical activity on most, if not all, days of the week. Avoid activities with a high risk of falling or abdominal trauma.
- *Breastfeeding women.* Be aware that neither acute nor regular exercise adversely affects the mother's ability to successfully breastfeed.
- *Older adults.* Participate in regular physical activity to reduce functional declines associated with aging and to achieve the other benefits of physical activity identified for all adults.

Food Groups to Encourage

Key Recommendations

- Consume a sufficient amount of fruits and vegetables while staying within energy needs. Two cups of fruit and 2.5 cups of vegetables per day are recommended for a reference 2,000-calorie intake, with higher or lower amounts depending on the calorie level.
- Choose a variety of fruits and vegetables each day. In particular, select from all five vegetable subgroups (dark-green, orange, legumes, starchy vegetables, and other vegetables) several times a week.
- Consume 3 or more ounce-equivalents of whole-grain products per day, with the rest of the recommended grains coming from enriched or whole-grain products. In general, at least half the grains should come from whole grains.

- Consume 3 cups per day of fat-free or low-fat milk or equivalent milk products.

Key Recommendations for Specific Population Groups

- *Children and adolescents.* Consume whole-grain products often; at least half the grains should be whole grains. Children 2 to 8 years should consume 2 cups per day of fat-free or low-fat milk or equivalent milk products. Children 9 years of age and older should consume 3 cups per day of fat-free or low-fat milk or equivalent milk products.

Fats

Key Recommendations

- Consume less than 10 percent of calories from saturated fatty acids and less than 300 mg/day of cholesterol, and keep *trans* fatty acid consumption as low as possible.
- Keep total fat intake between 20 to 35 percent of calories, with most fats coming from sources of polyunsaturated and monounsaturated fatty acids, such as fish, nuts, and vegetable oils.
- When selecting and preparing meat, poultry, dry beans, and milk or milk products, make choices that are lean, low fat, or fat free.
- Limit intake of fats and oils high in saturated and/or *trans* fatty acids, and choose products low in such fats and oils.

Key Recommendations for Specific Population Groups

- *Children and adolescents.* Keep total fat intake between 30 to 35 percent of calories for children 2 to 3 years of age and between 25 to 35 percent of calories for children and adolescents 4 to 18 years of age, with most fats coming from sources of polyunsaturated and monounsaturated fatty acids, such as fish, nuts, and vegetable oils.

Carbohydrates

Key Recommendations

- Choose fiber-rich fruits, vegetables, and whole grains often.
- Choose and prepare foods and beverages with little added sugars or caloric sweeteners, such as amounts suggested by the USDA Food Guide and the DASH Eating Plan.

- Reduce the incidence of dental caries by practicing good oral hygiene and consuming sugar- and starch-containing foods and beverages less frequently.

Sodium and Potassium

Key Recommendations

- Consume less than 2,300 mg (approximately 1 teaspoon of salt) of sodium per day.
- Choose and prepare foods with little salt. At the same time, consume potassium-rich foods, such as fruits and vegetables.

Key Recommendations for Specific Population Groups

- *Individuals with hypertension, blacks, and middle-aged and older adults.* Aim to consume no more than 1,500 mg of sodium per day, and meet the potassium recommendation (4,700 mg/day) with food.

Alcoholic Beverages

Key Recommendations

- Those who choose to drink alcoholic beverages should do so sensibly and in moderation—defined as the consumption of up to one drink per day for women and up to two drinks per day for men.
- Alcoholic beverages should not be consumed by some individuals, including those who cannot restrict their alcohol intake, women of childbearing age who may become pregnant, pregnant and lactating women, children and adolescents, individuals taking medications that can interact with alcohol, and those with specific medical conditions.
- Alcoholic beverages should be avoided by individuals engaging in activities that require attention, skill, or coordination, such as driving or operating machinery.

Food Safety

Key Recommendations

- To avoid microbial food-borne illness:
  - Clean hands, food contact surfaces, and fruits and vegetables. Meat and poultry should not be washed or rinsed.

- o Separate raw, cooked, and ready-to-eat foods while shopping, preparing, or storing foods.
- o Cook foods to a safe temperature to kill microorganisms.
- o Chill (refrigerate) perishable food promptly, and defrost foods properly.
- o Avoid raw (unpasteurized) milk or any products made from unpasteurized milk, raw or partially cooked eggs or foods containing raw eggs, raw or undercooked meat and poultry, unpasteurized juices, and raw sprouts.

Key Recommendations for Specific Population Groups

- *Infants and young children, pregnant women, older adults, and those who are immunocompromised.* Do not eat or drink raw (unpasteurized) milk or any products made from unpasteurized milk, raw or partially cooked eggs or foods containing raw eggs, raw or undercooked meat and poultry, raw or undercooked fish or shellfish, unpasteurized juices, and raw sprouts.
- *Pregnant women, older adults, and those who are immunocompromised.* Only eat certain deli meats and frankfurters that have been reheated to steaming hot.

2010 *DIETARY GUIDELINES FOR AMERICANS*

The 2010 *Dietary Guidelines for Americans* had 29 key recommendations, 23 of which are for the general population and 6 for specific population groups (USDA/HHS, 2010).

Balancing Calories to Manage Weight

Key Recommendations

- Prevent and/or reduce overweight and obesity through improved eating and physical activity behaviors.
- Control total calorie intake to manage body weight. For people who are overweight or obese, this will mean consuming fewer calories from foods and beverages.
- Increase physical activity, and reduce time spent in sedentary behaviors.
- Maintain appropriate calorie balance during each stage of life—childhood, adolescence, adulthood, pregnancy and breastfeeding, and older age.

Foods and Food Components to Reduce

- Reduce daily sodium intake to less than 2,300 mg and further reduce intake to 1,500 mg among persons who are 51 and older and those of any age who are African American or have hypertension, diabetes, or chronic kidney disease. The 1,500 mg recommendation applies to about half of the U.S. population, including children, and the majority of adults.
- Consume less than 10 percent of calories from saturated fatty acids by replacing them with monounsaturated and polyunsaturated fatty acids.
- Consume less than 300 mg per day of dietary cholesterol.
- Keep *trans* fatty acid consumption as low as possible by limiting foods that contain synthetic sources of *trans* fats, such as partially hydrogenated oils, and by limiting other solid fats.
- Reduce the intake of calories from solid fats and added sugars.
- Limit the consumption of foods that contain refined grains, especially refined grain foods that contain solid fats, added sugars, and sodium.
- If alcohol is consumed, it should be consumed in moderation—up to one drink per day for women and two drinks per day for men—and only by adults of legal drinking age.

Foods and Nutrients to Increase

Individuals should meet the following recommendations as part of a healthy eating pattern while staying within their calorie needs.

Key Recommendations

- Increase vegetable and fruit intake.
- Eat a variety of vegetables, especially dark-green and red and orange vegetables and beans and peas.
- Consume at least half of all grains as whole grains. Increase whole-grain intake by replacing refined grains with whole grains.
- Increase intake of fat-free or low-fat milk and milk products, such as milk, yogurt, cheese, or fortified soy beverages.
- Choose a variety of protein foods, which include seafood, lean meat and poultry, eggs, beans and peas, soy products, and unsalted nuts and seeds.
- Increase the amount and variety of seafood consumed by choosing seafood in place of some meat and poultry.
- Replace protein foods that are higher in solid fats with choices that are lower in solid fats and calories and/or are sources of oils.

- Use oils to replace solid fats where possible.
- Choose foods that provide more potassium, dietary fiber, calcium, and vitamin D, which are nutrients of concern in American diets. These foods include vegetables, fruits, whole grains, and milk and milk products.

Key Recommendations for Specific Population Groups

- Women capable of becoming pregnant should choose foods that supply heme iron, which is more readily absorbed by the body, additional iron sources, and enhancers of iron absorption such as vitamin C–rich foods.
- Women capable of becoming pregnant should consume 400 micrograms (mcg) per day of synthetic folic acid (from fortified foods and/or supplements) in addition to food forms of folate from a varied diet.
- Women who are pregnant or breastfeeding should consume 8 to 12 ounces of seafood per week from a variety of seafood types.
- Women who are pregnant or breastfeeding should limit white albacore tuna to 6 ounces per week and do not eat the following four types of fish: tilefish, shark, swordfish, and king mackerel due to their high methyl mercury content.
- Women, if pregnant, should take an iron supplement, as recommended by an obstetrician or other health provider.
- Individuals ages 50 years and older should consume foods fortified with vitamin B_{12}, such as fortified cereals or dietary supplements.

Building Healthy Eating Patterns

- Select an eating pattern that meets nutrient needs over time at an appropriate calorie level.
- Account for all foods and beverages consumed, and assess how they fit within a total healthy eating pattern.
- Follow food safety recommendations when preparing and eating foods to reduce the risk of food-borne illnesses.

2015–2020 *DIETARY GUIDELINES FOR AMERICANS*

The 2015–2020 *Dietary Guidelines for Americans* had 5 overarching guidelines and 13 supporting key recommendations (HHS/USDA, 2015).

5 Overarching Guidelines

1. Follow a healthy eating pattern across the life span.
2. Focus on variety, nutrient density, and amount.
3. Limit calories from added sugars and saturated fats, and reduce sodium intake.
4. Shift to healthier food and beverage choices.
5. Support healthy eating patterns for all.

13 Key Recommendations

- Consume a healthy eating pattern that accounts for all foods and beverages within an appropriate calorie level.

A healthy eating pattern includes

- A variety of vegetables from all of the subgroups—dark-green, red and orange, legumes (beans and peas), starchy, and other
- Fruits, especially whole fruits
- Grains, at least half of which are whole grains
- Fat-free or low-fat dairy, including milk, yogurt, cheese, and/or fortified soy beverages
- A variety of protein foods, including seafood, lean meats and poultry, eggs, legumes (beans and peas), and nuts, seeds, and soy products
- Oils

A healthy eating pattern limits:

- Saturated fats and *trans* fats, added sugars, and sodium

Key recommendations that are quantitative are provided for several components of the diet that should be limited. These components are of particular public health concern in the United States, and the specified limits can help individuals achieve healthful eating patterns within calorie limits:

- Consume less than 10 percent of calories per day from added sugars.
- Consume less than 10 percent of calories per day from saturated fats.
- Consume less than 2,300 milligrams (mg) per day of sodium.

- If alcohol is consumed, it should be consumed in moderation—up to one drink per day for women and up to two drinks per day for men—and only by adults of legal drinking age.

In tandem with the recommendations above, Americans of all ages—children, adolescents, adults, and older adults—should meet the *Physical Activity Guidelines for Americans* to help promote health and reduce the risk of chronic disease. Americans should aim to achieve and maintain a healthy body weight. The relationship between diet and physical activity contributes to caloric balance and managing body weight. As such, the *Dietary Guidelines* includes a key recommendation to:

- Meet the *Physical Activity Guidelines for Americans.*

REFERENCES

HHS/USDA (U.S. Department of Health and Human Services/U.S. Department of Agriculture). 2005. Dietary Guidelines for Americans, *2005.* Washington, DC: U.S. Government Printing Office. https://health.gov/dietaryguidelines/2005.asp (accessed July 24, 2017).

HHS/USDA. 2015. Dietary Guidelines for Americans *2015–2020: Eighth edition.* https://health.gov/dietaryguidelines/2015/guidelines (accessed July 24, 2017).

USDA/HHS. 1980. *Nutrition and your health:* Dietary Guidelines for Americans. *1st edition.* Washington, DC: U.S. Goverment Printing Office.

USDA/HHS. 1985. *Nutrition and your health:* Dietary Guidelines for Americans. *2nd edition.* Washington, DC: U.S. Government Printing Office. https://health.gov/dietaryguidelines/1985.asp (accessed July 24, 2017).

USDA/HHS. 1990. *Nutrition and your health:* Dietary Guidelines for Americans. *3rd edition.* Washington, DC: U.S. Government Printing Office.

USDA/HHS. 1995. *Nutrition and your health:* Dietary Guidelines for Americans. *4th edition.* Washington, DC: U.S. Government Printing Office.

USDA/HHS. 2000. *Nutrition and your health:* Dietary Guidelines for Americans. *5th edition.* Washington, DC: U.S. Government Printing Office.

USDA/HHS. 2010. Dietary Guidelines for Americans, *2010. 7th edition.* https://health.gov/dietaryguidelines/2010 (accessed July 24, 2017).

Appendix E

Additional Information About the Dietary Reference Intakes

The Dietary Reference Intakes (DRIs) are developed by committees that are independent of the process by which the *Dietary Guidelines for Americans* (*DGA*) are established. The DRIs provide a set of values describing the nutrient needs in apparently healthy populations. Although the values pertain to single nutrients, as opposed to foods and dietary patterns, the DRIs have played a key role in the evidence review of the Dietary Guidelines Advisory Committee (DGAC) and the recommendations in the *DGA Policy Report*. The DRIs underpin the *DGA* as the philosophy that if a person follows the recommendations of the *DGA Policy Report*, he or she will meet nearly all requirements as established by the DRIs (Britten et al., 2006). When DGAC conclusions change over time, food pattern modeling is applied to determine whether DRI values are still attainable. Given the interface between the DRIs and the *DGA*, the sections that follow provide context by presenting a historical perspective on the DRIs, outlining how the DRIs are intended to be used to assess nutritional adequacy and excesses, and describing the extent to which chronic disease end points have informed the DRIs.

A HISTORICAL PERSPECTIVE ON THE DIETARY REFERENCE INTAKES

Between 1941 and 1994, the Food and Nutrition Board (FNB) of what is now the National Academies of Sciences, Engineering, and Medicine issued 10 successive editions of the Recommended Dietary Allowances

(RDAs). As stated in the first of the reports, the RDAs were to act as a "guide to serve as a goal for good nutrition and as a 'yardstick' by which to measure progress toward that goal" (NRC, 1941, p. 1). These RDAs provided intake values for essential nutrients, which "were defined as chemical substances found in food that are necessary for human life and tissue growth and repair" (IOM, 1994, p. 8). RDA values were based, in large part, on prevention of the deficiency disease associated with lack of the specific essential nutrient, plus a margin of safety above this number to ensure good nutrition and protect all body tissues, termed "nutritional adequacy." Canada had a parallel process that produced values called Recommended Nutrient Intakes (RNIs) and resulted in recommendations similar to those put forth in the United States.

As science progressed, the RDA reports expanded the numbers of nutrients included and the types of biochemical end points used for establishing values. The RDAs also expanded to include both genders and all life stages. Concomitantly, there was a growing interest and emphasis on decreasing risk of chronic disease through diet, culminating in the report *Diet and Health: Implications for Reducing Chronic Disease Risk* (NRC, 1989), which in turn was based in part on two major secondary sources: *Surgeon General's Report on Nutrition and Health* and *Nutrition and Your Health: Dietary Guidelines for Americans* (HHS, 1988; USDA/HHS, 1985). *Diet and Health* addressed the science base for the relationship between nutrients, foods, and diet patterns and leading diet-related causes of morbidity and mortality in the United States at that time (NRC, 1989) (see Box E-1).

BOX E-1
Diet-Related Chronic Disease Included in the *Diet and Health* Report

- Atherosclerotic cardiovascular diseases (coronary heart disease, peripheral arterial disease, stroke)
- Cancer (esophageal, stomach, colorectal, liver, pancreatic, lung, breast, endometrial, ovarian, bladder, prostate)
- Dental caries
- Diabetes mellitus
- Hepatobiliary disease (cirrhosis of the liver, gallstones)
- Hypertension
- Obesity and eating disorders (anorexia, bulimia)
- Osteoporosis

SOURCE: NRC, 1989.

When *Diet and Health* was released, the FNB was in the process of determining whether to revise the tenth edition of the RDAs. There was a diversity of opinions as to "the challenge of whether to bring together the concepts of a health-promoting diet to reduce the risk of chronic disease and the nutrient-specific concepts underlying the RDAs" (IOM, 1994, p. 4). Ultimately, the FNB took a two-phase approach: (1) make a decision as to whether the RDAs should be revised; and (2) if so, determine the approach, strategy, and scope of work to revise them. To address the first phase, a public hearing was held in June 1993. One of the five questions posed to the speakers and audience was: "Should concepts of chronic disease prevention be included in the development of allowances?" (IOM, 1994, p. vi). At the end of the meetings, the speakers and testifiers unanimously agreed that it was time to revise the RDAs. The FNB produced a concept paper that summarized the symposium, public hearing, and discussions, stating:

> The science of human nutrition stands at a pivotal point in its development. We now understand not only that nutrients are essential for growth and development and health maintenance, but also that some play a role in the reduction of risk of chronic disease. (IOM, 1994, p. 1)

One of the conclusions from the concept paper states: "Reduction in the risk of chronic disease is a concept that should be included in the formulation of future RDAs where sufficient data for efficacy and safety exist" (IOM, 1994, p. 18)

In contrast to the previous RDA reports in the United States and RNI reports from Canada, in 1994 the two countries agreed to have one set of standards for both nations. The replacement and expansion of the RDAs and RNIs by the DRIs is a recognized key paradigm shift in how nutrient intakes are evaluated (IOM, 2006; Murphy et al., 2016). In addition to setting the values for determining nutrient adequacy, a new emphasis for the reference intakes was chronic disease prevention in apparently healthy populations. Another important difference in the new DRIs is the expansion of values (see Box 7-1). The introduction of the Estimated Average Requirements (EARs) value, for instance, allowed for progress toward making population-based recommendations. A collection of DRI reports have since been published and provide intake values for energy, macronutrients, and micronutrients (IOM, 1997, 1998, 2000a, 2001, 2005a,b, 2011). A variety of reports have also explored and explained how DRIs should be operationalized (IOM, 2000b, 2003a,b).

ASSESSING NUTRIENT ADEQUACY USING DIETARY REFERENCE INTAKE VALUES

The DRIs serve as a reference against which dietary intakes can be compared and can be used to assess the intakes of individuals. The current guidance for application of the DRIs indicates that the EAR, RDA, and Adequate Intake (AI) can be used to gauge the likelihood of usual dietary intake being adequate (IOM, 2000b). The evaluation of an individual's usual intake, however, "is imprecise and must be interpreted cautiously in combination with other types of information about the individual" (IOM, 2000b, p. 7).

Estimating the prevalence of inadequacy in groups requires different methods from those used for assessing individuals. The RDA, for instance, is not appropriate for the assessment of groups and should not be used. For nutrients with an EAR, the analysis can be performed using the probability approach or the EAR cut-point method. The probability approach has two key assumptions: (1) independence of intake and requirement, and (2) a known distribution of requirements (IOM, 2000b). This approach can be computationally challenging because it requires the selection of a probability model to properly execute. The EAR cut-point method is a shortcut to the probability approach and is performed by determining the proportion of the group with intakes below the EAR. This method typically provides similar results to the probability approach, and works particularly well when

> intakes are accurately measured, actual prevalence in the group is neither very low nor very high, estimated usual intakes of individuals are independent of each individual's requirements, the distribution of requirements is approximately symmetrical, and variability in intakes among individuals in the group is greater than the variability in requirements of the individual. (IOM, 2000b, p. 81)

Prevalence of nutrient inadequacy calculated using the EAR cut-point method can be underestimated or overestimated if one or more of the aforementioned assumptions are not met. Iron requirements do not meet the assumption of symmetry around the EAR, particularly in menstruating women, and use of the EAR cut-point method may lead to biased estimates of iron inadequacy (IOM, 2000b). An assessment of iron intake, especially among adolescent girls and premenopausal women, necessitates the use of the probability approach (IOM, 2000b). For nutrients with an AI, mean intake of a population meeting or exceeding the AI suggests prevalence of inadequacy is low.[1] The AI cannot, however, be

---

[1] Not all AIs are established based on indicators of inadequacy. Assessment of inadequacy in groups using such nutrients is made with less confidence.

used to determine the prevalence of inadequate nutrient intake for groups (IOM, 2000b).

ASSESSING RISK CAUSED BY EXCESSIVE INTAKES USING DIETARY REFERENCE INTAKE VALUES

The Tolerable Upper Intake Level (UL) does not represent an optimal or recommended intake level. Instead, it describes the highest intake level of a nutrient that is likely to pose little to no risk of a selected critical adverse effect for a given life stage and gender group. Table E-1 lists the adverse effects used to establish the existing ULs and demonstrates that values are largely not based on chronic disease end points or surrogate markers of chronic disease. Not all life stage groups or nutrients have a UL, which can make the assessment of excess consumption challenging. The rationale for not assigning a UL for saturated fat, for example, was that given the positive linear trends, "any incremental increase in saturated fatty acid intake increases [coronary heart disease] risk" (IOM, 2005a, p. 485).

INCLUSION OF CHRONIC DISEASE END POINTS IN DIETARY REFERENCE INTAKE VALUES

The vision for the DRIs was to include chronic disease risk reduction in the development of nutrition intake values as evidence emerged (IOM, 1994). The process for doing this has proven to be difficult. Determining a nutrient intake level that reflects the probability of developing a chronic disease does not operate the same way as the prevention of single nutrient deficiency conditions, because chronic diseases are multifactorial and absolute risk of a chronic disease in a given population is rarely 100 percent. Only five nutrients have nutritional adequacy DRI values that integrate chronic disease end points or surrogate markers of chronic disease (see Table E-2). Despite the complexities, efforts are currently under way to move toward using chronic disease end points to establish DRIs.[2]

[2] A multidisciplinary working group sponsored by the Canadian and U.S. government DRI steering committees met from late 2014 through April 2016 to consider how to base DRI values on chronic disease end points. The working group produced a report that provided extensive discussion of the issues and ideas for paths forward (Yetley et al., 2017). An ad hoc consensus committee of the National Academies of Sciences, Engineering, and Medicine recently released a report in which the options presented by Yetley et al. (2017) are reviewed and recommends methods and guiding principles for including chronic disease end points in the DRI process (NASEM, 2017).

TABLE E-1 Critical Adverse Effects Used to Establish Tolerable Upper Intake Levels in the Dietary Reference Intakes

Nutrient	Critical Adverse Effect Used to Establish Tolerable Upper Level
Boron[a]	Reproductive and developmental effects[b,c]
Calcium	Calcium excretion,[d] kidney stone formation[e,f,g]
Chloride[a]	Blood pressure status[h]
Choline[a]	Hypotension, fishy body odor[c,i]
Copper[a]	Liver damage[c]
Fluoride	Enamel and skeletal fluorosis
Folate[a,j]	Precipitating or exacerbating neuropathy in individuals deficient in B_{12}[c]
Iodine[a]	Elevated TSH concentration[c]
Iron	Gastrointestinal side effects
Magnesium[a,k]	Diarrhea and other gastrointestinal issues[f]
Manganese	Elevated blood concentrations and neurotoxicity[c]
Molybdenum[a]	Reproductive effects[b,c]
Niacin[a]	Flushing[f]
Nickel[a,l]	Decreased body weight gain[b,f]
Phosphorus[a]	Hyperphosphatemia[m,n,o,p]
Selenium	Hair and nail brittleness and loss
Sodium[a]	Blood pressure status[q]
Vanadium[r]	Renal toxicity[b]
Vitamin A	Teratogenicity,[s] liver abnormalities,[t] hypervitaminosis A[c,u]
Vitamin B_6[a,v]	Sensory neuropathy[c]
Vitamin C[a]	Osmotic diarrhea and related gastrointestinal disturbances[c]
Vitamin D	Hypercalcemia and related toxicity[w]
Vitamin E[a]	Hemorrhagic effects[b,c]
Zinc	Adverse effect on copper metabolism (i.e., reduced copper status)[x]

NOTES: Tolerable upper intakes levels are established based on intake of food, water, and supplements, unless otherwise noted. TSH = thyroid stimulating hormone.

[a] UL not determinable for infants ages 0 to 12 months.

[b] As observed in animal models.

[c] UL for children and adolescents (ages 1 to 18 years) were derived from the UL for adults.

[d] Used for infants.

[e] Used for adults.

[f] UL for children (ages 1 to 8 years) was derived from the UL for adults.

[g] UL for older children (ages 9 to 18 years) was derived from the UL for adults, with an additional amount added to account for metabolic demand increases and pubertal growth spurts.

TABLE E-1 Continued

[h] Chloride is assumed to be consumed in equimolar amounts as sodium. The UL, therefore, is the equimolar equivalent to the UL for sodium.

[i] Considered a secondary consideration.

[j] Limited to supplemental folate intake.

[k] UL is established for magnesium for nonfood sources.

[l] Derived from intake as soluble nickel salts.

[m] UL for adults (ages 19 to 70 years) was derived by dividing the approximate upper boundaries of normal serum inorganic phosphate levels in adults by an uncertainty factor.

[n] UL for toddlers and children (ages 1 to 8 years) was derived by dividing the approximate upper boundaries of normal serum inorganic phosphate levels in adults by a larger uncertainty factor than used for the adult UL, to account for the smaller body size.

[o] Because of the lack of evidence of a greater susceptibility of adverse effects, the UL for adolescents is the same as for adults.

[p] UL for older adults (ages > 70 years) was derived by dividing the approximate upper boundaries of normal serum inorganic phosphate levels in adults by a larger uncertainty factor than used for the adult UL, to account for increased prevalence of impaired renal function.

[q] UL for children (ages 1 to 18 years) was extrapolated from the UL for adults, based on estimated energy intakes.

[r] UL only determined for adults 19 years and older who are not pregnant or lactating.

[s] For women of childbearing age.

[t] For all other adults.

[u] Case reports in infants were used to derive a UL.

[v] UL for B_6 is based on evidence from oral supplemental doses of pyridoxine.

[w] UL for children (ages 1 to 8 years) was derived from the UL for adults. UL for older children and adolescents (ages 9 to 18 years) is the same as for adults.

[x] Because of a lack of available data, the UL for older infants, children, and adolescents were extrapolated from the UL for young infants.

SOURCES: IOM, 1997, 1998, 2000a, 2001, 2005b, 2011.

TABLE E-2 Nutritional Adequacy DRIs That Integrate Chronic Disease End Points and/or Surrogate Markers of Chronic Disease

Nutrient	Adequacy DRI Value(s)	Chronic Disease End Point
Calcium	EAR, RDA	Bone health (accretion, maintenance, and loss)[a]
Fluoride	AI	Dental caries
Potassium	AI	Combination of end points (salt sensitivity, kidney stones, blood pressure)
Total fiber	AI	Risk of coronary heart disease
Vitamin D	EAR, RDA	Bone health (accretion, maintenance, and loss)[b]

NOTES: The UL for sodium is based on blood pressure, which is considered a surrogate marker for chronic disease. Because the UL does not reflect a level of nutritional adequacy but rather represents an intake level after which risk of adverse effects increases, sodium in not included in this table. AI = Adequate Intake; DRI = Dietary Reference Intake; EAR = Estimated Average Requirement; RDA = Recommended Dietary Allowance.

[a] Measures varied by DRI life stage group and incorporated data on calcium balance, which is not directly linked to a specific chronic disease end point.

[b] Based on serum 25-hydroxyvitamin D concentrations to achieve bone health.

SOURCES: IOM, 1997, 2005a,b, 2011.

REFERENCES

Britten, P., K. Marcoe, S. Yamini, and C. Davis. 2006. Development of food intake patterns for the MyPyramid food guidance system. *Journal of Nutrition Education and Behavior* 38(6 Suppl):S78-S92.

HHS (U.S. Department of Health and Human Services). 1988. *The Surgeon General's report on nutrition and health.* Washington, DC: U.S. Government Printing Office. https://profiles.nlm.nih.gov/ps/access/nnbcqh.pdf (accessed May 15, 2017).

IOM (Institute of Medicine). 1994. *How should the Recommended Dietary Allowances be revised?* Washington, DC: National Academy Press.

IOM. 1997. *Dietary Reference Intakes for calcium, phosphorus, magnesium, vitamin D, and fluoride.* Washington, DC: National Academy Press.

IOM. 1998. *Dietary Reference Intakes for thiamin, riboflavin, niacin, vitamin B6, folate, vitamin B12, pantothenic acid, biotin, and choline.* Washington, DC: National Academy Press.

IOM. 2000a. *Dietary Reference Intakes for vitamin C, vitamin E, selenium, and carotenoids.* Washington, DC: National Academy Press.

IOM. 2000b. *Dietary Reference Intakes: Applications in dietary assessment.* Washington, DC: National Academy Press.

IOM. 2001. *Dietary Reference Intakes for vitamin A, vitamin K, arsenic, boron, chromium, copper, iodine, iron, manganese, molybdenum, nickel, silicon, vanadium, and zinc.* Washington, DC: National Academy Press.

IOM. 2003a. *Dietary Reference Intakes: Applications in dietary planning.* Washington, DC: The National Academies Press.

IOM. 2003b. *Dietary Reference Intakes: Guiding principles for nutrition labeling and fortification.* Washington, DC: The National Academies Press.

IOM. 2005a. *Dietary Reference Intakes for energy, carbohydrate, fiber, fat, fatty acids, cholesterol, protein, and amino acids*. Washington, DC: The National Academies Press.

IOM. 2005b. *Dietary Reference Intakes for water, potassium, sodium, chloride, and sulfate*. Washington, DC: The National Academies Press.

IOM. 2006. *Dietary Reference Intakes: The essential guide to nutrient requirements*. Washington, DC: The National Academies Press.

IOM. 2011. *Dietary Reference Intakes for calcium and vitamin D*. Washington, DC: The National Academies Press.

Murphy, S. P., A. A. Yates, S. A. Atkinson, S. I. Barr, and J. Dwyer. 2016. History of nutrition: The long road leading to the Dietary Reference Intakes for the United States and Canada. *Advances in Nutrition: An International Review Journal* 7(1):157-168.

NASEM (National Academies of Sciences, Engineering, and Medicine). 2017. *Guiding principles for developing Dietary Reference Intakes based on chronic disease*. Washington, DC: The National Academies Press.

NRC (National Research Council). 1941. *Recommended Dietary Allowances*. Washington, DC: National Academy Press.

NRC. 1989. *Diet and health: Implications for reducing chronic disease risk*. Washington, DC: National Academy Press.

USDA/HHS (U.S. Department of Agriculture). 1985. *Nutrition and your health:* Dietary Guidelines for Americans. 2nd ed. Washington, DC: U.S. Government Printing Office. https://health.gov/dietaryguidelines/1985.asp (accessed May 15, 2017).

Yetley, E. A., A. J. MacFarlane, L. S. Greene-Finestone, C. Garza, J. D. Ard, S. A. Atkinson, D. M. Bier, A. L. Carriquiry, W. R. Harlan, D. Hattis, J. C. King, D. Krewski, D. L. O'Connor, R. L. Prentice, J. V. Rodricks, and G. A. Wells. 2017. Options for basing Dietary Reference Intakes (DRIs) on chronic disease endpoints: Report from a joint US-/Canadian-sponsored working group. *American Journal of Clinical Nutrition* 105(1):249S-285S.

Appendix F

Committee Member and Staff Biographies

COMMITTEE MEMBERS

Robert M. Russell, M.D. (*Chair*), is professor emeritus of Medicine and Nutrition at Tufts University. Dr. Russell has served on many national and international advisory boards including the U.S. Department of Agriculture Human Investigation Committee (Chairman), the U.S. Food and Drug Administration, U.S. Pharmacopoeia Convention, National Institutes of Health (NIH), the World Health Organization, UNICEF, and the American Board of Internal Medicine. He has worked on international nutrition programs in several countries including China, Guatemala, Haiti, Iran, Iraq, the Philippines, and Vietnam. Dr. Russell is a member of numerous professional societies, on the editorial boards of four professional journals, a past president of the American Society for Nutrition (ASN), and is now President of the ASN Foundation. Dr. Russell co-edited two editions of *Present Knowledge in Nutrition* and was the Editor in Chief of *Nutrition Reviews*. Dr. Russell served as a member of the National Academy of Sciences panels on Folate, Other B Vitamins, and Choline, and as chair of the panel on Micronutrients. He is a National Associate of the National Academies of Sciences, Engineering, and Medicine (the National Academies). He is former chair of the Food and Nutrition Board (FNB) of the National Academies, and is a fellow of ASN. Dr. Russell presently is working with the Biomarkers of Nutrition for Development (BOND) Program of NIH and is on the board of Haiti Projects. He also has recently served as a board member of the Nestlé and Fetzer Foundations. He has received numerous national and international awards for his research on retinoids and carotenoids (Kritchevsky, Atwater, DSM awards), and has authored more than 300 scientific papers and 5 books. He received his M.D. from Columbia University.

Jamy Ard, M.D., is a professor in the Department of Epidemiology and Prevention and in the Department of Medicine at Wake Forest University Baptist Medical Center. He is also co-director of the Wake Forest Baptist Health Weight Management Center, directing medical weight management programs. Dr. Ard received an M.D. and completed internal medicine residency training at Duke University Medical Center. He also received formal training in clinical research as a fellow at the Center for Health Services Research in Primary Care at the Durham Veterans Affairs Medical Center. Dr. Ard has more than 15 years of experience in clinical nutrition and obesity. Prior to joining the faculty at Wake Forest in 2012, Dr. Ard spent 9 years at The University of Alabama at Birmingham (UAB) where he served as medical director of UAB's EatRight Weight Management Services, vice chair for clinical care in the Department of Nutrition Sciences, and associate dean for clinical affairs in the School of Health Professions. Dr. Ard's research interests include clinical management of obesity and strategies to improve cardiometabolic risk using lifestyle modification. He has been conducting research on lifestyle modification since 1995 and has worked on several NIH-funded multicenter trials, including Dietary Approaches to Stop Hypertension (DASH), DASH-sodium, and Weight Loss Maintenance Trial. His work has been published in numerous scientific journals, and he has been a featured presenter at several conferences and workshops dealing with obesity. Dr. Ard has served on several expert panels and guideline development committees, including the Institute of Medicine Committee on Consequences of Sodium Reduction in Populations, the American Heart Association/American College of Cardiology/The Obesity Society Guideline Panel on the Identification, Evaluation, and Treatment of Overweight and Obesity in Adults, and currently, the American Psychological Association Obesity Guideline Development Panel. He is also serving on the editorial board for the *American Journal of Clinical Nutrition* and the *International Journal of Obesity*.

Stephanie A. Atkinson, Ph.D., D.Sc. (Hon.), is a professor and nutrition clinician–scientist, Department of Pediatrics, associate member, Department of Biochemistry and Biomedical Sciences, Faculty of Health Sciences, McMaster University, and professional staff in McMaster Children's Hospital, Hamilton. A key focus of her research has been investigations of the factors influencing skeletal development in premature and term infants and in children with boney morbidity secondary to disease process and/or drug therapy (particularly steroids) in diseases such as lymphoblastic leukemia, nephrosis, rheumatoid disorders, cystic fibrosis, or epilepsy. Her current research encompasses clinical trial and epidemiological investigations of the environmental (nutrition), genetic, and biochemical factors during fetal, neonatal, and early childhood life that play a role in defining the offspring phenotype and as risk determinants for noncommunicable diseases. She leads a multidisciplinary team of researchers in the conduct of randomized clinical intervention trials of nutrition and exercise in pregnancy designed to optimize maternal and child health outcomes including bone health. Dr. Atkinson served on the Scientific Oversight Committee for the Dietary Reference Intakes (DRIs) from 1995 to 2004 and several DRI projects and workshops since that time. Most recently she has served as a working group member for the DRI and Chronic Diseases Endpoints project cosponsored by Health Canada and the Office of Dietary Supplements of NIH. Dr. Atkinson currently serves as chair of the Board of Directors of the Maternal, Infant, Child and Youth Health Research Network (MICYRN) and colead of the MICYRN Canadian Birth Cohort Coalition to harmonize data from Canadian birth cohort studies, as Executive Member of Board of Trustees of the North American International Life Sciences Institute (Washington, DC), and as a member of the Scientific Advisory Council for Osteoporosis Canada. Dr. Atkinson is an elected Fellow of both the American Society for Nutrition and the Canadian Academy of Health Sciences and was recently awarded a Doctor of Science, honoris causa, from Western University in London, Canada.

Carol J. Boushey, Ph.D., M.P.H., R.D., is the director of the Nutrition Support Shared Resource at the University of Hawaii Cancer Center. Her research has involved working as part of multidisciplinary teams, which is crucial for providing support to the member investigators of the Cancer Center as they design and conduct studies that include the collection and analyses of dietary intake and other nutritional issues. She specializes in the broad spectrum of evaluating dietary exposures with an emphasis on use of technology and assessing diverse racial/ethnic groups. In collaboration with scientists in engineering at Purdue University, she created the Technology Assisted Dietary Assessment program that uses image analysis and visualization on small mobile devices (e.g., mobile telephones), to aid researchers in collecting dietary intake with limited burden. She has been fundamental in describing dietary intakes of several Pacific Northwest Tribal Nations and young children in jurisdictions in the Pacific. Dr. Boushey is actively involved with the dietary assessment methods used with the Multiethnic Cohort (MEC), which includes 215,000 adults representing five ethnic groups (Japanese, Hawaiian, non-Hispanic white, African American, Hispanic/Latino). As a member of the Dietary

Patterns Methods Project, she completed analyses in the MEC showing that consuming a dietary pattern that achieves a high diet-quality index score is associated with lower risk of mortality from all causes, cardiovascular disease, and cancer in adult men and women. She has been the chief architect of paper- and computer-based dietary assessment methods to assess calcium consumption among Asian, Hispanic, and non-Hispanic white adolescents in the United States. Dr. Boushey received her Ph.D. from the University of Washington and her M.P.H. from the University of Hawaii at Manoa.

Susan M. Krebs-Smith, Ph.D., M.P.H., is the chief of the Risk Factor Assessment Branch of the Epidemiology and Genomics Research Program (EGRP) in the National Cancer Institute's Division of Cancer Control and Population Sciences (DCCPS). She oversees EGRP's research portfolio and initiatives that focus on the development, evaluation, and dissemination of high-quality risk factor metrics, methods, tools, technologies, and resources for use across the cancer research continuum, as well as the assessment of cancer-related risk factors in the population. Her own surveillance research has emphasized trends in intake of foods and nutrients, especially fruits and vegetables; food sources of nutrients; and factors associated with the intake of foods and/or nutrients, using data from the National Nutrition Monitoring and Related Research Program. Her contributions in the area of dietary assessment methodology have focused on developing methods to assess dietary patterns and the usual intake of foods. Her efforts in dietary guidance and food policy include quantifying potential future demand for food commodities based on population-wide adoption of the *Dietary Guidelines for Americans* and census projections. Dr. Krebs-Smith provided data analyses and consultation in support of the last several editions of the *Dietary Guidelines for Americans* and was a member of the Institute of Medicine's Committee to Develop a Framework for Assessing the Effects of the Food System. Prior to joining EGRP, Dr. Krebs-Smith was the chief of the Risk Factor Monitoring and Methods Branch in the Applied Research Program (now the Health Care Delivery Research Program), DCCPS. She received her Ph.D. from the Pennsylvania State University and her M.P.H. from the University of Minnesota.

Joseph Lau, M.D., is professor emeritus in the Center for Evidence Synthesis in Health within the School of Public Health at Brown University and was the co-director of the Agency for Healthcare Research and Quality (AHRQ) designated Evidence-based Practice Center (EPC) at Brown. Prior to Brown, he was a professor of medicine and professor of clinical and translational science at the Institute for Clinical Research and Health

Policy Studies at Tufts Medical Center. He directed the Tufts EPC from 1997 until 2012 and led the production of more than 80 evidence reports, technology assessments, and comparative effectiveness reviews under contract with the AHRQ. He has served as a member of an FDA advisory committee, and as a member of a Food and Agriculture Organization of the United Nations/World Health Organization workshop. He served as a member on two Institute of Medicine committees including Framework to Evaluate the Safety of Dietary Supplements and Standards for Clinical Practice Guidelines. He received his M.D. from Tufts University School of Medicine and completed a fellowship in clinical decision making and medical computer science at the New England Medical Center.

Bruce Y. Lee, M.D., M.B.A., is an associate professor of international health at the Johns Hopkins Bloomberg School of Public Health, executive director of the Global Obesity Prevention Center (GOPC) at Johns Hopkins, and director of operations research at the International Vaccine Access Center (IVAC) as well as associate professor at the Johns Hopkins Carey Business School. Dr. Lee has more than 15 years of experience in industry and academia in systems science and developing and implementing mathematical and computational methods, models, and tools to assist decision making in public health and medicine. He has been the Principal Investigator for projects supported by a variety of organizations and agencies including the Bill & Melinda Gates Foundation, NIH, AHRQ, the Centers for Disease Control and Prevention (CDC), UNICEF, the Global Fund, and the U.S. Agency for International Development. His previous positions include serving as Senior Manager at Quintiles Transnational, working in biotechnology equity research at Montgomery Securities, cofounding Integrigen, and serving as an associate professor at the University of Pittsburgh, where he founded PIHCOR (Public Health Computational and Operations Research), which is now based at Johns Hopkins. Dr. Lee has authored more than 180 scientific publications (including more than 90 first author and more than 35 last author) as well as 3 books: *Principles and Practice of Clinical Trial Medicine*, *What If…?: Survival Guide for Physicians*, and *Medical Notes: Clinical Medicine Pocket Guide*. He is an associate editor for the journal *Vaccine* and deputy editor for *PLOS Neglected Tropical Diseases*. He is a regular contributor to *The Huffington Post* and *Forbes*. He and his work have garnered attention in leading media outlets such as *The New York Times*, *Los Angeles Times*, *Time*, *CBS News*, *Businessweek*, *U.S. News & World Report*, *Bloomberg News*, *Reuters*, and National Public Radio (NPR). Dr. Lee received his B.A. from Harvard University, his M.D. from Harvard Medical School, and his M.B.A. from the Stanford Graduate School of Business. He completed his internal medicine residency training at the University of California, San Diego.

Joanne R. Lupton, Ph.D., is a distinguished professor emerita at Texas A&M University, where she was a faculty member for 31 years prior to retiring in 2015. She chaired the Macronutrients Panel for the Dietary Reference Intakes that determined the intake values for protein, carbohydrates, fats, fiber, and energy for the United States and Canada and she also chaired the Institute of Medicine panel to determine the definition of dietary fiber. She was a member of the 2005 U.S. Dietary Guidelines Advisory Committee. She is currently serving a second term on FNB. Dr. Lupton spent 1 year at FDA helping to develop levels of scientific evidence required for health claims. While there she was appointed to the Commissioner's Task Force for Better Nutrition and received a Commissioner's Special Citation for her work. She was elected to the National Academy of Medicine in 2010 and is a lifetime associate of the National Academy of Sciences. Dr. Lupton has mentored more than 100 M.S. and Ph.D. students while at Texas A&M, and received the Dannon/American Society for Nutrition mentoring award in 2004. In 2007 she received the Texas A&M University distinguished achievement award for research. In 2010 she received the ASN General Mills Bell Institute of Health and Nutrition–Innovation Award. Dr. Lupton is Past President of ASN, the nutrition research organization. Her research is on the effect of diet on colon physiology and colon cancer with a particular focus on dietary fiber and n-3 fatty acids. She has received the Vahouny Medal for her research on dietary fiber. She translates basic research on diet and colon physiology to science-based public policy and has consulted with individuals in China, Japan, South Korea, Taiwan, and elsewhere on the definition of dietary fiber and establishing dietary guidance systems in those countries. Her undergraduate degree is from Mt. Holyoke College, and her Ph.D. in nutrition is from the University of California, Davis.

Sally C. Morton, Ph.D., is the dean of the College of Science at Virginia Tech, and holds the Lay Nam Chang Dean's Chair. Her research focuses on evidence synthesis and patient-centered comparative effectiveness research. Previously, Dr. Morton served as chair of the Department of Biostatistics in the Graduate School of Public Health and director of the Comparative Effectiveness Research Center at the University of Pittsburgh, vice president for statistics and epidemiology at RTI International, and head of the RAND Corporation Statistics Group. Dr. Morton was president of the American Statistical Association (ASA) and chair of Section U (Statistics) of the American Association for the Advancement of Science, and she is a fellow of both organizations. She is a member of the Patient-Centered Outcomes Research Institute Methodology Committee, and the AHRQ EPCs Program Methods Steering Committee. She has served on several National Academies committees, the Census Scientific Advisory

Committee, and the National Academies Committee on National Statistics. Dr. Morton holds a Ph.D. in statistics from Stanford University.

Nicolaas P. Pronk, Ph.D., is the president of the HealthPartners Institute and Chief Science Officer at HealthPartners and holds a faculty appointment as Adjunct Professor of Social and Behavioral Sciences at the Harvard T.H. Chan School of Public Health in Boston, Massachusetts. Dr. Pronk's work is focused on connecting evidence of effectiveness with the practical application of programs, practices, policies, and systems that measurably improve population health and well-being. His research interests include workplace health and safety, obesity, physical activity, and systems approaches to population health and well-being. Currently, Dr. Pronk serves as a co-chair of the U.S. Secretary of Health and Human Services' Advisory Committee on National Health Promotion and Disease Prevention Objectives for 2030 (Healthy People 2030) and is a member of the Community Preventive Services Task Force. He was the founding and past president of the International Association for Worksite Health Promotion and has served on boards and committees at the National Academies; the American Heart Association; and the Health Enhancement Research Organization, among others. He is widely published in both the scientific and practice literatures with more than 400 articles, books, and book chapters and is an international speaker on population health and health promotion. Dr. Pronk received his doctorate degree in exercise physiology at Texas A&M University and completed his postdoctoral studies in behavioral medicine at the University of Pittsburgh Medical Center at the Western Psychiatric Institute and Clinic in Pittsburgh, Pennsylvania.

Susan B. Roberts, Ph.D., is the director of the Energy Metabolism Laboratory, professor of nutrition and co-director of the Obesity Research Cluster in the Jean Mayer Human Nutrition Research Center on Aging at Tufts University, and professor of psychiatry and scientific staff member in pediatrics in the Tufts University School of Medicine. She received her Ph.D. from the University of Cambridge, United Kingdom, and did postdoctoral training at the Massachusetts Institute of Technology before moving to Tufts in 1987. Her research focuses on determinants of weight regulation, including dietary composition factors such as glycemic index, protein, and fiber, and behavioral factors in weight control. In addition to her work in the United States she has conducted studies in Brazil, China, The Gambia, Guinea Bissau, and the United Kingdom. She has published more than 240 research papers in research journals, including the *New England Journal of Medicine* and *JAMA*, and has an H-index of 61. Dr. Roberts was the 2009 awardee of the E.V. McCollum award of the American Society for Nutrition to recognize the creativity and importance of her work on weight regulation, and the 2016 W.O. Atwater Lecturer for important contributions to nutrition and health worldwide.

A. Catharine Ross, Ph.D., is a professor and the occupant of the Dorothy Foehr Huck Chair of Nutrition in the Department of Nutritional Sciences at The Pennsylvania State University. As a nutritional biochemist, Dr. Ross has studied cellular factors involved in the biosynthesis and transport of vitamin A molecules. Her focus has been on the interaction of cellular retinoid-binding proteins and enzymes that esterify retinol for transport, storage, and oxidation with the intent to link biochemical findings with nutritional studies to better understand how vitamin A homeostasis is regulated by dietary status and metabolic conditions. She also investigates the role of retinoids in immune function, principally antibody production. Dr. Ross has received numerous awards, including the Mead-Johnson Award and the Osborne and Mendel Award from the American Society for Nutrition. She is active within a range of professional societies, including the American Association of Immunologists, Sigma Xi, and the American Physiological Society, and has served on a number of committees for the American Society for Nutrition and the Federation of the American Societies for Experimental Biology. Dr. Ross is a fellow of the American Association for the Advancement of Science and a member of the National Academy of Sciences. She chaired the committee on Dietary Reference Intakes for Vitamin D and Calcium and served on the FNB panel on Micronutrients for the Dietary Reference Intakes, and the committee on Opportunities in the Nutrition of Food Sciences. Dr. Ross is also a member of FNB. Dr. Ross received her Ph.D. from Cornell University in biochemistry and molecular and cell biology.

Barbara O. Schneeman, Ph.D., served as the higher education coordinator for the U.S. Agency for International Development (USAID). In this role, Dr. Schneeman worked with the higher education community to improve awareness of USAID opportunities and increase engagement avenues for the agency. Previously she served as the director of the Office of Nutrition, Labeling, and Dietary Supplements at FDA from 2004 to 2013. In that position, she oversaw the development of policy and regulations for dietary supplements, labeling, food standards, infant formula, and medical foods, and she served as U.S. delegate to two Codex committees (Food Labeling and Nutrition and Foods for Special Dietary Uses). From 1976 to 2004, she was a member of the nutrition faculty at University of California, Davis, and is currently emeritus professor of nutrition. She has been a visiting scientist at University of California, San Francisco, and Assistant Administrator for Nutrition in the Agricultural Research Service of USDA. Professional activities include participation in Dietary Guidelines Advisory Committees (1990 and 1995) and FNB of the National Academies, among others. She is recognized for her work on dietary fiber, gastrointestinal function, and policy development in the area of food and nutrition. She received her B.S. degree in food science from the University of California, Davis; her Ph.D. in nutrition from the University of California, Berkeley; and her postdoctoral training in gastrointestinal physiology at Children's Hospital in Oakland, California.

Martín J. Sepúlveda, M.D., FACP, FAAP, FACOEM, is an IBM Fellow and elected member of the National Academy of Medicine. He is recently retired from the IBM Corporation where he had a distinguished career, serving in numerous executive capacities including vice president of Health Systems and Policy Research and vice president of Integrated Health Services. He led health policy, strategy, health benefits, services and operations, occupational health, and well-being for IBM globally. He is widely recognized for contributions in public and population health, private-sector health care, wellness, and health benefits innovation. He led private-sector collaboration with clinicians for medical home transformation leading to formation of the Patient-Centered Primary Care Collaborative. Dr. Sepúlveda received his M.D. and M.P.H. degrees from Harvard University, his B.A. magna cum laude from Yale University, and he completed residencies in internal medicine at UCSF Hospitals, and occupational/environmental medicine at the National Institute for Occupational Safety and Health. He trained in the Epidemic Intelligence Service of the Centers for Disease Control and Prevention, and completed a fellowship in internal medicine at the University of Iowa Hospitals and Clinics. He serves on several boards including the American Board of Internal Medicine Foundation, The New York Academy of Medicine, and the Council for Health Research for Economic Development.

STAFF

Samantha M. Chao is a senior program officer at the National Academies. Previously she was a manager at The Pew Charitable Trusts where she developed and implemented a process to ensure the integrity and quality of research produced by teams across almost 30 policy areas. In that role, she advised teams on design and conduct of high-quality research methods at the national, state, and local levels. At Pew she also worked on the State Health Care Spending project to enumerate the cost of health care to states. Prior to joining Pew, she directed numerous studies at the National Academies, including the groundbreaking report *Health IT and Patient Safety*. She focused primarily on health care quality, performance measures, payment models, and methods to improve the quality and value of health care through the strengthening of research. She also conducted studies related to the U.S. Social Security Administration, integrative medicine, and continuing education for health professionals. She completed an M.P.H. in health policy with a concentration in management at the University of Michigan.

Meghan E. Quirk is a senior program officer on FNB. Dr. Quirk's current projects include working with a committee to develop a workshop on federal, state, tribal, and local strategies to limit sugar-sweetened beverages among young children and assisting on a study to review the process for updating the *Dietary Guidelines for Americans*. Dr. Quirk has also worked on the recently completed review of the Special Supplemental Nutrition Program for Women, Infants, and Children (WIC) food packages and directed a study on interpreting reports on obesity prevalence and trends. Prior to joining the National Academies, Dr. Quirk was a postdoctoral research associate at Tennessee State University where she gained experience in community-based participatory research. She was part of a collaborative team that developed a smartphone app designed to provide nutrition education information to families with a preschool-aged child enrolled in WIC. She earned her doctorate from Emory University, where her research focused on the clinical and dietary evaluation of patients prescribed a newly approved drug for the management of phenylketonuria. During her graduate training, she was also involved in efforts to develop nutritional management guidelines of five inborn errors of metabolism. She earned her bachelor's degree in nutrition and dietetics from the University of New Mexico.

Anna Bury is a research associate at the National Academies. She is jointly supporting the consensus study that is reviewing the process to update the *Dietary Guidelines for Americans*, and the Food Forum, a longstanding initiative of the FNB. During her time at the National Academies, she has assisted with two additional consensus studies, *Assessing Prevalence and Trends in Obesity: Navigating the Evidence*, and *Finding a Path to Safety in Food Allergy: Assessment of the Global Burden, Causes, Prevention, Management, and Public Policy*. She received her bachelor's degree in public health and sustainable development from Gordon College, where her research focused on the relationship between sustainable agricultural systems and community health, with case studies in Morocco, Switzerland, and the United States.

Meredith J. Young joined FNB as a Senior Program Assistant in September 2016. She is jointly supporting the consensus study that is reviewing the process to update the *Dietary Guidelines for Americans* and a workshop titled *Strategies to Limit Sugar-Sweetened Beverage Consumption in Young Children*. Prior to joining the National Academies, she worked at Virginia Polytechnic Institute and State University as a health education office assistant and an undergraduate research assistant. She has experience supporting clinical research, specifically controlled feeding studies assessing the effects of prebiotic supplementation and cocoa supplementation in pre-diabetic adults, the effects of high-sugar diets in children, and the effects of high-fat feeding in college-aged males. She received her bachelor's degree in human nutrition, foods, and exercise with a concentration in dietetics from Virginia Polytechnic Institute and State University.

Ann L. Yaktine is the director of FNB of the National Academies. FNB applies scientific knowledge to advise the nation on policies related to food, nutrition, and food safety, and their roles in health maintenance and disease prevention. In her role as director, she is responsible for developing, implementing, and managing the board's activities, as well as engaging FNB members in strategic planning to identify important and emerging issues in nutrition, food sciences, and food safety. Dr. Yaktine is a 2008 recipient of the Institute of Medicine's Cecil Award. In 2009 she participated in the Korea-U.S. Symposium on the Science of Food Safety Assessment. She has published journal reports on nutrition and cancer, nutrients and contaminants in foods, and nutrition assistance programs. Dr. Yaktine is a member of the Academy of Nutrition and Dietetics and the American Society for Nutrition. She holds a master's degree in nutrition from the University of Kansas and a Ph.D. in biochemistry and cancer biology from the Eppley Institute for Research in Cancer and Allied Diseases at the University of Nebraska Medical Center.

Appendix G

Disclosure of Conflicts of Interest

The conflict-of-interest policy of the National Academies of Sciences, Engineering, and Medicine (www.nationalacademies.org/coi) prohibits the appointment of an individual to a committee like the one that authored this Consensus Study Report if the individual has a conflict of interest that is relevant to the task to be performed. An exception to this prohibition is permitted only if the National Academies determine that the conflict is unavoidable and the conflict is promptly and publicly disclosed.

When the committee that authored this report was established a determination of whether there was a conflict of interest was made for each committee member given the individual's circumstances and the task being undertaken by the committee. A determination that an individual has a conflict of interest is not an assessment of that individual's actual behavior or character or ability to act objectively despite the conflicting interest.

Dr. Jamy Ard was determined to have a conflict of interest because in addition to his academic appointments, he serves as medical director for a medical food-based program that is owned by a company in the food industry.

Dr. Susan Roberts was determined to have a conflict of interest because she serves as chief scientific advisor and shareholder of a weight management company.

Dr. Barbara Schneeman was determined to have a conflict of interest because she serves on two scientific advisory councils in the food and agriculture industries.

In each case, the National Academies determined that the experience and expertise of the individuals were needed for the committee to accomplish the task for which it was established. The National Academies could not find other available individuals with the equivalent experience and expertise who did not have conflicts of interest. Therefore, the National Academies concluded that the conflicts were unavoidable and publicly disclosed them through the National Academies Current Projects System (www8.nationalacademies.org/cp).